THE MEDICAL GUIDE for Dentists Treating Complex Patients

Leslie S.T. Fang, MD, PhD
Tracey Wong Menhall, MSc

THE MEDICAL GUIDE

for Dentists Treating Complex Patients

edra
PUBLISHING

This edition first published 2025

ISBN 9781962679909
eISBN 9781962679473

Books Editor in Chief: Paola Sammaritano, Edra S.p.A.
Books Project Manager: Sandra A. Calarota, Edra S.p.A.
Cover and Layout: Barbara Rastelli

edra
PUBLISHING

Edra Publishing US LLC
3309 Northlake Boulevard,
Suite 203,
Palm Beach Gardens,
FL 33403
EIN: 844113980
info@edrapublishing.com
www.edrapublishing.com

Printed in Italy in March 2025 by RGM Printing, Bergamo

TABLE OF CONTENTS

PHARMACOLOGY AND THE DENTIST

CARDIOVASCULAR DISEASE

ENDOCRINE DISORDERS

RESPIRATORY DISEASES

HEPATIC DISORDERS

RENAL DISORDER

HEMATOLOGY

ONCOLOGY

INFECTIOUS DISEASE

CENTRAL NERVOUS SYSTEM DISORDER

PSYCHIATRIC DISORDER

RHEUMATOLOGIC DISORDER

PREGNANT PATIENT

NURSING MOTHER

SEDATION DENTISTRY

1 MEDICAL HISTORY AND FOCUSED PHYSICAL EXAMINATION RELEVANT TO THE DENTAL MANAGEMENT OF THE MEDICALLY COMPROMISED PATIENT

IMPORTANCE OF THE MEDICAL HISTORY

As enormous progress is being made in both medicine and dentistry, a thorough but focused medical history and physical examination are important in the optimal care of the patient. Dentistry now encompasses procedures that can last hours and significant use of local anesthetics with vasoconstrictors and sometimes with sedation. This would pose stress to the patient in the chair, particularly if they have medical comorbidities. It is critical that all new patients have a careful documentation of their medical history.

It is also critical to stress that, whenever you need additional information that the patient may not have, it is prudent to get the information from the patient's physician. It is sometimes necessary to get medical clearance for dental procedures from the patient's physician, particularly if sedation is involved.

The medical history can be in the form of a fill-in form self-reported by the patient. The form needs to be customized according to the dental practice and the types of dental intervention most commonly encountered in the practice. Figure 1.1 represents an abbreviated medical history form.

Although a very simple inquiry, this will help identify potential risks, particularly with respect to lengthy intervention in the patient with medical comorbidities.

1. Patient demographics

- Date of birth
- Age
- Gender and gender identification
- Height
- Weight
- Marital status
- Profession

2. Medical history

Every practice will have to decide the kind of details they would like to incorporate into the form they use on all new patients. For every section of the form, a subsequent chapter will detail the dental evaluation and dental management. Some of the questions asked will be clarified in these chapters.

Since it is a self-report by the patient, some of the details might well be missing. If deemed important, missing information should be sought from the patient's physician.

The following represents the most comprehensive information that one might want, and one should modify the form one needs according to the type of practice one has. In general, one should start off with a simple form **(Figure 1.1)** and use the following information to drill in on the details.

FIGURE 1.1 A sample short patient questionnaire

Last name				
First name				

Gender		Male	Female	Other
Date of birth				
Marital status				
Height				
Weight				
Profession				

Cardiovascular disease		Yes	No	Comment
	Hypertension	Yes	No	
	Coronary artery disease	Yes	No	
	Myocardial infarction	Yes	No	
	Arrhythmia	Yes	No	
	Congestive heart failure	Yes	No	
	Cardiac intervention	Yes	No	
	Coronary intervention (stent, etc.)	Yes	No	
	Cardiac devices (pacemaker, etc.)	Yes	No	

Diabetes mellitus		Yes	No	
	Type 1	Yes	No	
	Type 2	Yes	No	
	Diabetic complications	Yes	No	

Cancer		Yes	No	
	Type of cancer			
	Surgery	Yes	No	
	Chemotherapy	Yes	No	
	Radiation therapy	Yes	No	
	Cancer in remission	Yes	No	

Pulmonary diseases		Yes	No	
	Asthma	Yes	No	
	COPD	Yes	No	

Liver diseases		Yes	No	
	History of hepatitis	Yes	No	
	History of cirrhosis	Yes	No	
	History of non-alcoholic steatohepatitis (fatty liver)	Yes	No	

Gastrointestinal diseases		Yes	No	
	Gastroesophageal reflux	Yes	No	
	Inflammatory bowel disease	Yes	No	
	Irritable bowel syndrome	Yes	No	

Renal disease		Yes	No	
	Chronic kidney disease Stage II III IV V (circle appropriate stage)			

Thyroid disease		Yes	No	
	Hypothyroidism	Yes	No	
	Hyperthyroidism	Yes	No	
	Thyroid cancer	Yes	No	

Adrenal disease		Yes	No	
	Cushing's disease	Yes	No	
	Adrenal insufficiency	Yes	No	

Hematologic disease		Yes	No	
	Bleeding disorder	Yes	No	
	Anticoagulation therapy	Yes	No	
	Anti-platelet therapy	Yes	No	
	Anemia	Yes	No	
	Leukemia	Yes	No	

Neurological disease		Yes	No	
	Transient ischemic attack	Yes	No	
	Stroke	Yes	No	

Psychiatric disorder		Yes	No	
	Generalized anxiety disorder	Yes	No	
	Depression	Yes	No	

SOCIAL HISTORY

	Smoking history	Yes	No	___ packs per day for ___ years
	Alcohol intake	Yes	No	Average ___ drinks per week
	Other drug use	Yes	No	Type of drug use
	Exercise	Yes	No	Average ___ hours per week

FAMILY HISTORY

	Mother	Alive	Deceased	
	Father	Alive	Deceased	
	Siblings	Alive	Deceased	

MEDICATIONS

Prescribed medications	Name	Dose

Over-the-counter medications	Name	Dose

Supplements and nutraceuticals	Name	Dose

Allergies	Name	Type of allergy

Based upon the responses in the sample history and medication form, one can then focus on the positive responses and ask additional questions for the details relevant to dentistry.

Details of medical history

- **Cardiovascular history**
  - Hypertension
  - Coronary artery disease
    - Angina
    - Myocardial infarction
  - Percutaneous coronary intervention
    - Angioplasty
    - Atherectomy
    - Stents
      - Bare metal stents
      - Drug eluting stents
      - Bioresorbable scaffolds
  - Coronary artery bypass surgery
    - Number of vessels bypassed
    - Type of bypass
  - Valvular intervention
    - Open heart surgery for valvular replacement
    - Transcatheter valvular interventions
  - Arrhythmia
    - Atrial fibrillation
    - Supraventricular tachycardia
    - Ventricular arrhythmia
    - Heart blocks
  - Congestive heart failure
    - Ejection fraction, if known
    - Functional classification (New York Heart Association Classification, if known)
  - Implant devices
    - Permanent pacemaker
    - Defibrillator
    - Watchman device

- **Diabetes mellitus**
  - Type 1 or type 2?
  - Diabetic complications:
    - Renal insufficiency
    - Retinopathy
    - Neuropathy
    - Periodontal disease
    - Infections, particularly oral infections
  - Most recent HbA1c
  - Glucose monitoring devices
  - Insulin pump

- **Cancer**
  - Type of cancer
  - Chemotherapy and inclusive dates
  - Radiation therapy and inclusive dates
  - Head and neck radiation
  - Current status of cancer

- **Pulmonary diseases**
  - Asthma
  - Chronic obstructive pulmonary disease
  - Interstitial lung disease
  - Pulmonary fibrosis
  - History of CO_2 retention
  - History of oxygen dependence

- **Hepatic diseases**
  - History of hepatitis
    - Hepatitis A
    - Hepatitis B
      - Acute
      - Chronic carrier

- Hepatitis C
  - Chronic carrier
  - Treated and cured
- Non-alcoholic steatohepatitis
- Treatment of hepatitis
  - Conservative management
  - Medications used in treatment
  - Current status after treatment
- Cirrhosis
  - Etiology of cirrhosis
  - Stage of cirrhosis
  - Severity of cirrhosis
  - History of variceal bleeding
  - History of hepatic encephalopathy
- Treatment of cirrhosis
  - Conservative management
  - Medications
  - Liver transplant

- **Gastrointestinal diseases**
  - Peptic ulcer disease
  - Inflammatory bowel disease
  - Irritable bowel syndrome

- **Renal disease**
  - Chronic kidney disease (Stage I–V)
    - Etiology of CKD, if known
    - Electrolyte derangement
    - Acid base balance
    - Hypertension
    - Fluid overload and congestive heart failure
  - Dialysis
    - Type of dialysis
      - Hemodialysis
      - Peritoneal dialysis
      - Home dialysis
    - Days of dialysis
    - Anticoagulation use
  - Renal transplant
    - Living related transplant
    - Living unrelated transplant
    - Cadaveric transplant

- **Thyroid disease**
  - Hypothyroidism
  - Hyperthyroidism
  - Thyroid cancer
  - Thyroid surgery
  - Thyroid radiation therapy

- **Adrenal disorder**
  - Adrenal insufficiency
  - Adrenal hormone excess
  - Chronic steroid use

- **Hematologic disorders**
  - Anemia
    - Etiology
    - Treatment
  - Platelet disorder
  - Anticoagulation therapy
  - Hematologic malignancies

- **Bone disorders**
  - Osteoporosis
  - Multiple myeloma

- **Neurological disorders**
  - Seizures
  - Transient ischemic attacks
  - Cerebrovascular accidents

- **Psychiatric disorders**
  - Depression
  - Generalized anxiety disorder
  - History of alcohol excess
    - Number of glasses of alcohol consumed per week
    - History of hospitalization for detoxification
  - History of substance abuse

3. Medications

In the form, leave plenty of room for patients to fill in their medications.

- All prescribed medication and dosage
- All over-the-counter medications
- All supplements and nutraceuticals

This will give you a very quick view of the medical complexity of the patient you are treating.

This information will also guide you to avoid potential drug-drug interactions of drugs you may be prescribing. For instance, a course of antibiotics for odontogenic infections may prolong PT/INR in a patient on coumadin.

A complete list of ALL medications is particularly important if the dental procedure involves sedation.

4. Physical examination

It is important to do an abbreviated physical examination and a detailed oral examination.

Vital signs

- BP
- Pulse
- Weight
- Height
- Oxygen saturation if deemed appropriate (e.g., for sedation dentistry)

Detailed oral examination

Examination of the dentition and evaluation of lumps and sores.

Oral lesions that should be sought for are included in Chapter 2.

5. Review of system

An abbreviated review will help flag potential ongoing issues that may interfere with optimal dental care of the patient.

6. Family history

Special attention should be paid to family history of cardiovascular disease, strokes and, in particular, bleeding diathesis.

7. Social history

- Marital status
- Current or previous job
- Smoking history
- Alcohol intake
- Drug use
- Exercise
- Sexual preference

8. Laboratory results

Laboratory results may play an important role in the dental management of the patient. The pertinent laboratory results will be discussed in greater detail in each of the chapters. In general, these tests are ordered by the patient's physician, but the relevant results should be incorporated into the patient's record.

2

DIAGNOSIS OF ORAL DISEASE

IMPORTANCE OF THE ORAL EXAMINATION

The diagnosis and management of oral lesions are two of the most rewarding and challenging services the dental practitioner can provide. The oral examination should be part of every dental visit. The initial evaluation should be detailed, and evaluation on subsequent visits can be more focused.

There are a finite number of oral lesions that the dental practitioner should master:

- White lesions
- Ulcerations
- Vesicles
- Tumors
- Pigmented lesions

1. Focused history

Oral lesions may be incidentally found during a routine examination. Alternatively, the patient may have a specific complaint at presentation.

For patients presenting with a complaint of an oral lesion, careful evaluation of the history is of great importance. The patient should be allowed to describe the presenting symptoms without leading questions:

- Symptoms
    - The most common symptom is that of pain
    - Swelling
    - Roughness of the mucosa
    - Bleeding
    - Pigmentation

- Onset of symptoms
    - Acute onset favors inflammation and are rarely neoplastic
    - Chronic lesions progressing slowly is less likely to be inflammatory in nature
- Duration of symptoms
- Distribution of lesions
    - Local lesions
    - Bilateral lesions
    - Systemic manifestations such as allergy or viral infections
    - Are there systemic signs associated with the lesions: fevers, malaise, lymphadenopathy)?
- Clinical course
    - Is the lesion healing?
    - Is the lesion progressing?
    - Is the lesion not changing?
- Exogenous modifiers
    - Trauma?
    - Drug related?
    - Smoking history
    - Recent contact with sick patients
    - Foreign travel
    - Recent dental care

2. Clinical examination

The clinical examination on the initial visit should include a complete head and neck examination. Although the patient may have specific concerns, it is still important to have a complete examination. One should do the oral examination in an orderly manner. In addition to the oral examination, blood pressure, pulse and, in specific circumstances, the pulse oximetry should be routinely checked and recorded.

Based upon the responses in the sample history and medication form, one can then focus on the positive responses and ask additional questions for the details relevant to dentistry.

Intraoral examination

- Lips
- Buccal mucosa
- Labial mucosa
- Hard palate
- Soft palate
- Oral pharynx
- Tongue
- Floor of the mouth
- Salivary glands

Extraoral examination

- Facial symmetry
- Jaw
- Nose
- Ears
- Eyes
- Skin
- Cervical areas

3. Adjunctive techniques for a diagnosis

Biopsy

Biopsies can be performed in the dental office with local anesthetics.

Hemostasis can be accomplished by direct pressures, sutures or placement of a periodontal pack.

- Incisional biopsy: small portion of the lesion is obtained
- Excisional biopsy: lesion totally excised

Specimens should be submitted under preservation to a qualified laboratory.

Post-operative infection is rare with biopsies.

Exfoliative cytology

- The area of interest is gently stroked by the tip of a wet wooden tongue depressor
- Cellular debris is smeared evenly on a glass microscope slide
- Placed in a fixative of alcohol and ether
- The preparation is submitted to a qualified laboratory

Immunofluorescence

Immunofluorescence testing, using sera and biopsies, may play an important role in the diagnosis and assessment of autoimmune diseases.

- Pemphigus vulgaris
- Pemphigoid
- Lichen planus
- Systemic lupus erythematosus

There are services that will provide test kits that facilitate immunofluorescence testing. The services provide, at no cost, containers for biopsies of mucosa to be sent for immunofluorescence testing to a qualified laboratory.

4. Diagnosis of the lesions

White lesions

White coloration is caused by the collection of dead cells, bacteria and debris on the tissue surface. There are two kinds of white lesions in the oral cavity:

- **Necrotic lesions**
  - Candidiasis
    - Nystatin suspension 200,000–400,000 U TID for 14 days
    - Clotrimazole 10 mg troches five times a day for 14 days
    - Fluconazole 400 mg day 1, 200 mg QD for 14 days
  - Burns
    - White necrotic lesion related to epithelial sloughing
    - Usually easy to diagnose on the basis of history
- **Keratotic lesions**

  The coloration of keratotic lesion is attributed to the presence of excessive keratin.
  - **Hyperkeratosis**
    - Caused by chronic irritation of the oral mucosa
    - May occur anywhere in the mouth but are most common on the buccal mucosa and on the lateral borders of the tongue
    - Smoking aggravates hyperkeratosis
    - No treatment is necessary
  - **Leukoplakia**
    - White plaques
    - Consequence of chronic irritation
    - Should eliminate source of irritation
    - Biopsy if lesions persist
    - 7% of patients with leukoplakia demonstrate histologic evidence of dysplasia or carcinoma
  - **Lichen planus**
    - Etiology unclear
    - An inflammatory autoimmune condition
    - Often have skin lesions as well in the flexor surfaces of the arms and legs
    - Histologically, lesions are characterized by an extensive submucosal T-cell and mast cell infiltration
  - **White sponge nevus**
    - Benign, genetically inherited keratotic condition that affects the mouth and other mucosal surfaces
    - Asymptomatic
    - Bilateral, raised spongy hyperkeratotic lesion
    - No treatment necessary
  - **Systemic lupus erythematosus**
    - Oral lesions in 40% of patients
    - Most common oral lesion is hyperkeratosis.
    - Can also present with ulcers and vesiculobullous lesions
    - Often present in conjunction with skin lesions

Oral cancers

Oral cancers are uncommon and accounts for less than 3% of new cancers.

- **Risk factors**
    - ❑ Tobacco is a major risk factor in the development of oral cancer
    - ❑ Alcohol also contributes risk in the development of oral cancer
    - ❑ Evidence of genetic predisposition
    - ❑ Contribution of viral infection
    - ❑ Contribution of immunological factors
- **Appearance**
    - ❑ Appears as a nonhealing, painless and expanding ulcer on any mucosal surface
    - ❑ The most common sites are the lateral or ventral edge of the posterior tongue
- **Diagnosis**
    - ❑ Clinical observation and palpation
    - ❑ Biopsy
    - ❑ Cytology

Ulcers

- **Recurrent aphthous stomatitis**

  The most common ulcer in the oral cavity is **recurrent aphthous stomatitis.**
    - ❑ Recurrent lesions every few months
    - ❑ May be associated with systemic conditions such as Behcet's syndrome, vitamin B_{12} and folate deficiency, HIV, inflammatory bowel disease
    - ❑ May be associated with infections such as HIV, syphilis, tuberculosis, viral infection and mucormycosis
- **Acute necrotizing ulcerative gingivitis**
    - ❑ ANUG is a fusospirochetal infection of the gingiva
    - ❑ Abrupt onset of localized or diffuse gingiva pain
    - ❑ Acute gingival bleeding
    - ❑ Bad taste and fetor odor
    - ❑ 50% of patients experience systemic manifestation of infection, including fever, malaise and lymphadenopathy
    - ❑ Localized or generalized areas of papillary and marginal necrosis that start interproximally and spread laterally
    - ❑ The areas of necrosis produce a pseudomembrane that overlies an inflammatory base
    - ❑ Loss of the interdental papilla causes a "punched out" appearance
    - ❑ Tissue is friable and bleeds easily
    - ❑ Treatment with penicillin
    - ❑ Gentle debridement after infection and inflammation are controlled

Vesiculobullous lesions

- Small, fluid filled blisters on the mucosa
- Usually ovoid
- Often related to autoimmune diseases
- Causes:
  - **Pemphigus vulgaris**
    - Most serious of the oral blistering diseases
    - Genetic alteration
    - Causes severe, chronic, progressive vesiculobullous lesions
    - Epidermal sloughing
    - Histologically, presence of anti-desmosomal antibodies resulting in destruction of the substance that cements epithelial cells together. Intraepithelial separation of the stratum germinativum from the underlying stratum spinosum results in acantholysis
  - **Mucous membrane pemphigus**
    - Initially bullous lesion that progresses to erosion
    - Gingiva is almost always affected with desquamative gingivitis
    - Lesions are very painful
    - Lesions are aggravated by removable prosthesis
    - Secondary surface infection is common
    - Diagnosis by biopsy with immunofluorescent studies
    - May involve the conjunctiva
  - **Bullous pemphigus**
    - Skin is the usual primary site of involvement
    - Fewer than 20% of patients with bullous pemphigus have oral bullous lesions
    - Oral lesions involve the gingiva, appearing like desquamative gingivitis
  - **Lichen planus**
    - Most commonly appear as white keratotic lesions
    - However, it can present as bullous lesions as well
    - Present as painful desquamative gingivitis
    - Responds to topical steroids
  - **Erythema multiforme**
    - Acute mucocutaneous disease as a result of an immune complex deposition
    - Often has an explosive onset
    - Skin lesions have characteristic target appearance
    - Etiology unclear but often follows infection such as herpes, mycoplasma or fungi

  - Can be caused by a wide variety of drugs
  - Diagnosed by history of acute onset and appearance of the lesions
  - Biopsy is usually not necessary
- **Certain drug eruption**

  Virtually any drug can potentially cause drug eruption.
  - Analgesics
  - Antibiotics
  - Anticonvulsants
  - Antituberculous drugs
  - Antidiabetic drugs
  - Antineoplastic drugs
  - Antihypertensive drugs
  - Antirheumatic drugs
  - Psychopharmacologic agents

Pigmented lesions

- Most common mucosal pigmentation is related to melanin
- Less common etiology of mucosal pigmentation related to bilirubin and iron
- Excessive melanin deposition can be seen in:
  - Addison's disease
  - Peutz-Jeghers syndrome
  - Melanoma
  - Endocrine disorders

3 THE MOST COMMONLY PRESCRIBED MEDICATIONS IN DENTISTRY

INTRODUCTION

There are many drugs that can be prescribed in dentistry, and the type of practice and the type of patients in the practice may dictate individual prescribing protocols. However, it is important to master a small number of medications that you may use frequently. In general, antibiotics, analgesics and narcotics constitute the bulk of the prescriptions written by the dental professionals.

1. Antibiotics

Antibiotics are commonly prescribed in dentistry. The proper deployment of antibiotics for premedication and for treatment of odontogenic infections is detailed in Chapters 6, 7, 8 and 10. The use of antibiotics around the time of implant placement is discussed in Chapter 11.

In general, the emphasis is to avoid excessive use of antibiotics and to use the least amount of appropriate antibiotics for the shortest duration necessary. In general, the use of clindamycin is to be minimized. These recommendations are to address the increasing concerns over antibiotic resistance and adverse effects of antibiotics.

While there are unique circumstances where special antibiotics may be appropriate, the seven most commonly prescribed antibiotics in **Table 3.1** would represent >90% of the clinical situations where antibiotics are prescribed in dentistry.

Because of the unique composition of the oral flora, penicillin-based antibiotics remain one of the most frequently prescribed medication in dental practices. Although penicillin VK is still prescribed, its dosing schedule (QID) results in the more common use of amoxicillin and amoxicillin-clavulonic acid.

TABLE 3.1 Antibiotics commonly prescribed

Amoxicillin	500 mg TID or 875 mg BID
Amoxicillin-clavulonic acid	500 mg TID or 875 mg BID
Azithromycin	500 mg day 1 250 mg days 2 to 5 or 500 mg QD for 3 days
Cephalexin	500 mg QID Do not use in patients with angioedema, urticaria or anaphylaxis to penicillin or amoxicillin
Clindamycin	300 mg QID Its use is gradually being phased out
Metronidazole	500 mg TID
Ciprofloxacin	500 mg BID

Both amoxicillin and amoxicillin-clavulonic acid can be dosed as 875 mg BID, which is more convenient for the patient resulting in higher compliance. Amoxicillin-clavulonic acid is generally prescribed in instances where there is concern over anaerobic infection. Clindamycin has been the mainstay of antibiotics for premedication and treatment of odontogenic infection in penicillin-allergic patients. It is gradually being replaced because of concerns over C. *difficile* colitis and development of drug-resistant organisms. When used, it is generally prescribed in a 300 mg QID regimen.

Cephalexin is now increasingly proposed for patients with a history of penicillin allergic reactions. However, there is a small chance of cross-reactivity (5-29%) with penicillin with immediate reaction. It should therefore not be prescribed for patients whose penicillin allergy involved angioedema, urticaria or anaphylaxis. It is generally prescribed in a 500 mg QID regimen.

Azithromycin is a good alternative for patients with a penicillin allergy. It does not have as good an anaerobic coverage. It is prescribed as 500 mg on day 1 and 250 mg from days 2 to 5. Alternatively, it can be prescribed as 500 mg QD for 3 days. Azithromycin has been reported to cause QTc prolongation in rare instances. This can potentially result in lethal arrhythmias. Use of azithromycin should be carefully reviewed in elderly patients, particularly those with pre-existing arrhythmias or those that are already on medications that can cause QTc prolongation.

Although clarithromycin is a macrolide similar to azithromycin, its metabolism by CYP3A4 leads to drug-drug interactions not seen with azithromycin. Its dosing schedule 500 mg BID also makes it less convenient than azithromycin. In general, one should use azithromycin whenever a macrolide is considered. Clarithromycin can also cause, although rarely, QTc prolongation.

In instances where additional anaerobic coverage is important, metronidazole can be added at 500 mg TID. Metronidazole should be added to existing aerobic coverage and should not be used as a standalone drug. Patients prescribed metronidazole should be warned to completely abstain from alcohol since metronidazole has an *Antabuse* (disulfiram) effect.

In instances where coverage for sinus organisms is desired (e.g., sinus lift procedures), ciprofloxacin at 500 mg BID can be prescribed. Ciprofloxacin can also cause QTc prolongation in rare instances, with its attendant cardiovascular risks. It should be prescribed judiciously to elderly patients, patients with pre-existing arrhythmias or patients already on drugs that can cause QTc prolongation.

2. Analgesics

In general, acetaminophen should be the foundation for pain control and non-steroidal anti-inflammatory drugs can be added to synergize its efficacy. The proper use of analgesics and anti-inflammatory drugs is detailed in Chapter 3.

For mild pain, acetaminophen is the most logical analgesic to use. Acetaminophen can be administered in doses of 650 mg every 4 hours or 1,000 mg every 8 hours.

It is important not to exceed 3,000 mg per day. In instances where there is concern over hepatic function, the dose should be reduced by one half to not exceed 1,500 mg per day.

In instances where additional analgesia is desired, non-steroidal anti-inflammatory drugs can be added to acetaminophen **(Table 3.2)**.

TABLE 3.2 Commonly prescribed analgesics and anti-inflammatory drugs

Drug	Dose
Acetaminophen	650 mg Q6H or 1,000 mg Q8H
Ibuprofen	600 mg QID or 800 mg TID
Naproxen	550 mg BID
Celecoxib	400 mg first dose Then 200 mg BID for no more than 3 days

Non-steroidal anti-inflammatory drugs can cause gastrointestinal irritation. They are contraindicated in patients with pre-existing renal insufficiency since it can precipitate acute kidney injury.
Ibuprofen can be given in doses of 600 mg QID or 800 mg TID.
Naproxen can be given in doses of 550 mg BID.
Celecoxib can be given in doses of 100 mg BID. For management of severe pain, celecoxib can be prescribed in a regimen with 400 mg as a first dose, followed by 200 mg BID for no more than 3 days.

3. Opioids

Opioid use in dentistry **(Table 3.3)** has drawn scrutiny and should be reserved for the rare instances where one cannot get adequate pain control at maximal doses of analgesics and anti-inflammatory drugs. Most studies in dental pain control have indicated that the efficacy of acetaminophen plus high-dose non-steroidal anti-inflammatory drugs is equivalent to or superior to that of narcotics.
Acetaminophen should be added to the narcotic to optimize efficacy. Although commercially available combinations of acetaminophen and narcotics are commonly prescribed, one should get used to prescribing acetaminophen separately from the opioids. This would permit more careful titration of opioid use.

TABLE 3.3 Commonly prescribed narcotics

Oxycodone	5 mg Q4-6H or 7.5 mg Q4-6H or 10 mg Q4-6H
Hydrocodone	5 mg Q4-6H or 7.5 mg Q4-6H or 10 mg Q4-6H
Tramadol	100 mg load then 50 mg Q4H

In general, one ought to be comfortable with the use of these 14 medications, which should constitute 90% of medications prescribed. The specific deployment of these medications in the different dental situations will be discussed in Chapters 6, 7, 8, 9, 10, 11 and 12.
Pediatric dosing of these medications is discussed in Chapter 13.

4 COMMONLY PRESCRIBED ANALGESICS AND ANTI-INFLAMMATORY DRUGS

INTRODUCTION

Pain control after dental procedures and pain control for patients with an active odontogenic infection are important aspects of patient care. It is important to stress that most dental pain can be controlled by analgesics in combination with anti-inflammatory drugs, with results similar to or superior to the use of narcotics. The goal of pain management in dentistry is to minimize the need for use of narcotics in these settings.

It is important to choose medications that are most appropriate for the level of pain anticipated.

1. Pre-emptive analgesia

Increasingly, it is recognized that if one can give analgesics and anti-inflammatory drugs prior to the occurrence of pain, it will minimize pain after the procedure. The principle is to control pain prior to the emergence of pain. Once pain is allowed to emerge, it will take considerably higher doses of analgesics and anti-inflammatory drugs to suppress the pain.

It is therefore reasonable to administer analgesics and anti-inflammatory drugs just prior to the procedure.

To optimize patient compliance, one should prescribe medications with longer half-lives. For instance, naproxen and celecoxib are preferred over ibuprofen.

Acetaminophen 1000 mg together with +/- naproxen 550 mg would be a good pre-emptive regimen in instances where post-operative pain is anticipated.

2. Analgesics for mild pain

In general, acetaminophen should be the foundation for pain control, and non-steroidal anti-inflammatory drugs can be added to synergize its efficacy.

For mild pain, acetaminophen is the most logical analgesic to use **(Table 4.1)**. Acetaminophen can be administered in doses of 650 mg every 4 hours or 1,000 mg every 8 hours.

It is important not to exceed 3,000 mg per day. In instances where there is concern over hepatic dysfunction, the dose should be reduced by one half to not exceed 1,500 mg per day. In most instances, acetaminophen alone would suffice for the control of mild pain. In some instances, non-steroidal anti-inflammatory drugs might be added to augment the analgesic.

TABLE 4.1 Analgesics for mild pain

Pre-emptive analgesics pre-operatively	
Acetaminophen 650 mg Q4H or Acetaminophen 1000 mg Q8H	Not to exceed 3,000 mg per day Less than 1,500 mg in patients with liver disease

3. Analgesics and anti-inflammatory for moderate pain

In instances where moderate pain is anticipated, non-steroidal anti-inflammatory drugs should be added to acetaminophen to get the synergistic effect for pain control (Table 4.2).
Ibuprofen can be given in doses of 600 mg QID or 800 mg TID.
Naproxen can be given in doses of 550 mg BID.
Celecoxib can be given in doses of 400 mg as a single dose, followed by 200 mg BID for no more than 3 days.

TABLE 4.2 Analgesics and anti-inflammatory drugs for moderate pain

Pre-emptive analgesic and anti-inflammatory drugs pre-operatively	
Ibuprofen	600 mg QID or 800 mg TID
Naproxen	550 mg BID
Celecoxib	400 mg first dose Then 200 mg BID for no more than 3 days

4. Management of severe pain

Pre-emptive analgesics and anti-inflammatory drugs should be administered pre-operatively.
Post-operatively, analgesics in combination with non-steroidal anti-inflammatory drugs should be given at maximal doses at least for the first 24-48 hours. If one can prevent pain from emerging, it would minimize the need for narcotics in this small population with severe pain after dental procedure.
If narcotics are necessary, the dental professional should follow the policies and recommendations for prescribing opioids recommended in Chapter 5.
In general, one ought to be comfortable with pre-emptive analgesia, which is currently underutilized. One should be treating expected pain aggressively with a combination of acetaminophen and anti-inflammatory drugs to minimize the use of narcotics for pain control.

5 POLICIES AND RECOMMENDATIONS FOR PRESCRIBING OPIOIDS IN THE MANAGEMENT OF DENTAL PAIN

INTRODUCTION

There is concern that opioids may be prescribed excessively in dentistry. It is clear that in the majority of the instances, pain can be controlled with the combination of analgesics and anti-inflammatory drugs without invoking the need for opioids.
When prescribing opioids, it is important to be mindful of the recommended guidelines.

1. Opioids for severe pain

In the rare instances where pain cannot be adequately controlled by analgesics and anti-inflammatory drugs, opioids may be added to optimize pain control.
Opioids commonly prescribed generally belong to the families of codeine, hydrocodone or oxycodone. Table 5.1 shows the bio-equivalency of the five families of medications. Rarely, tramadol or meperidine are used.
In general, these opioids are added to acetaminophen or non-steroidal anti-inflammatory drugs to optimize efficacy.

TABLE 5.1 Bio-equivalency of the five commonly prescribed opioids

Bio-equivalency	
Codeine	45 mg
Hydrocodone	7.5 mg
Oxycodone	5 mg
Meperidine	100 mg
Tramadol	100 mg

2. Combination drugs

There are many drugs combining opioids with either acetaminophen or non-steroidal anti-inflammatory drugs to optimize efficacy in pain control (Table 5.2). It is expected that these combinations will be gradually phased out since one can easily forget the exact amounts of the component parts and run the risk of over-prescription of opioids. It is therefore prudent to prescribe the opioid separately from the analgesics and anti-inflammatory drugs.

For severe pain, combinations may include acetaminophen or anti-inflammatory drugs added to opioids.

TABLE 5.2 Commonly prescribed opioids and maximal dosing

Commonly prescribed opioids (given Q4-6H)			
Ultram	100 mg tramadol load Then 50 mg Q4H		
Norco 7.5	7.5 mg hydrocodone	325 mg APAP	MAX 9 per day
Vicodin, Vicodin ES	5 mg hydrocodone 7.5 mg	300 mg APAP	MAX 10 per day
Percocet 5, 7.5	5, 7.5 mg oxycodone	325 mg APAP	MAX 9 per day
Tylenol #3	30 mg codeine	300 mg APAP	MAX 10 per day
Tylenol #4	60 mg codeine	300 mg APAP	MAX 10 per day
Add NSAID* or Celebrex (Celecoxib) to one of the above			
Vicodin HP	10 mg hydrocodone	300 mg APAP	MAX 10 per day
Norco 10	10 mg hydrocodone	325 mg APAP	MAX 9 per day
Percocet 10	10 mg oxycodone	325 mg APAP	MAX 9 per day
Demerol	50 mg meperidine		Q4-6H

* Non-steroidal anti-inflammatory drug.

3. Understanding the amount of opioids prescribed

Because different doses of the different opioids have different efficacy, it is useful to convert what one is prescribing in terms of equivalency of morphine as expressed as milligrams of morphine prescribed (Table 5.3).

It is suggested that whenever an opiate is to be prescribed that the clinician convert the prescribed dose to the morphine milligram equivalent so as to be able to see how the prescribed dose compares to morphine.

TABLE 5.3 Gauging efficacy by comparing equivalency to morphine

Morphine milligram equivalency	
Morphine	1
Hydrocodone	1
Oxycodone	1.5
Codeine	0.15
Meperidine	0.10
Tramadol	0.10

4. Policies and recommendations for prescribing opioids

Different governing bodies have different policies and recommendations for prescribing opioids. In general, these are designed to optimize patient safety, to minimize unnecessary prescription of opioids and to minimize the possibility of drug addiction and abuse. Most of the governing bodies have mandated continuing education certification for prescribers.

Implementation of these policies and recommendations have significantly decreased the prescription of opioids with little compromise in pain control.

Many governing bodies have implemented the need for prescribers to enroll in a prescription drug monitoring program. This program tracks all opioids prescribed to any given patient over the course of the past few years. This would allow the prescriber to have immediate information about the patient's history of opioid use and would drastically decrease the likelihood of promoting addiction and abuse.

In general, one should always prescribe the lowest effective dose: Determining the morphine milligram equivalence allows for more precise and knowledgeable dosing.

For dental pain, one should prescribe no greater quantity than needed for the expected duration of pain, which is usually 3 days.

One should never prescribe opioids for longer than 7 days.

The ultimate goal is to ensure patient safety and comfort while minimizing the use of opioids.

6 LOCAL ANESTHETICS AND VASOCONSTRICTORS

INTRODUCTION

Local anesthetics with vasoconstrictors are uniformly employed in dental procedures. One should be comfortable with the use of agents most relevant to one's practice.
It is important not to exceed the maximal allowance per dose of local anesthetic or vasoconstrictors in any patient in any given session.
Specific medical concerns may lead to changes in administration, particularly with respect to the limitation of vasoconstrictors in patients with cardiovascular concerns.

1. Types and maximal dose of local anesthetics

There are five basic forms of local anesthetics, each with a different onset and duration of action. It is important to master specific agents that are most relevant for one's specific type of practice **(Table 6.1)**.
All five local anesthetics are in the amide family. Articaine is structurally different in that it contains an ester group and has a thiophene instead of a benzene ring. In some studies, articaine was more likely to achieve successful anesthesia than lidocaine.
Lidocaine is a local anesthetic with a fast onset of action and short duration of action. It is the most commonly used for local anesthetics.
In specific instances where a long duration of action is desired, bupivacaine may be administered.

TABLE 6.1 Types of local anesthetics

Generic	Brand name	Onset	Duration
Lidocaine	Xylocaine	2-4 min	60-90 min
Articaine	Septocaine	2-4 min	60-220 min
Mepivacaine	Carbocaine	2-4 min	90-180 min
Prilocaine	Citanest	2-4 min	90-220 min
Bupivacaine	Marcaine	5-8 min	180-440 min

While using local anesthetics, it is important to adhere to the maximal doses allowed in order not to get into issues with toxicity. Local anesthetic systemic toxicity can result in central nervous system and cardiovascular toxicity.
In a 70 kg person, the maximal numbers of carpules of the different local anesthetics are estimated in Table 6.2.

TABLE 6.2 Maximal one-time dose of local anesthetic*

Lidocaine 2%	13 carpules
Articaine 4%	7 carpules
Mepivacaine 2%	11 carpules
Mepivacaine 3%	7 carpules
Prilocaine 4%	8 carpules
Bupivacaine 0.5%	10 carpules

*Estimated for a 70 kg person.

It is important to stress that the maximal one-time dose of local anesthetic is also predicated on the maximal one-time dose of vasoconstrictors present in the local anesthetic-vasoconstrictor combination.

2. Types and maximal one-time dose of vasoconstrictors

Vasoconstrictors are used in combination with local anesthetics in dentistry. Vasoconstrictors allow for concentration of the local anesthetics in a confined area, maximizing the efficacy and duration of the local anesthetics while minimizing the systemic absorption. It also contributes to hemostasis.

Epinephrine and levonordefrin, in varying concentrations, are available in combination with local anesthetics. It is important to stay below the maximal allowable one-time dose of vasoconstrictors **(Table 6.3)**.

TABLE 6.3 Maximal one-time dose of vasoconstrictor*

Epinephrine 1:50,000	5.5 carpules
Epinephrine 1:100,000	5.5–11 carpules
Epinephrine 1:200,000	5.5–11 carpules
Levonordefrin 1:20,000	11 carpules

*Estimated for a 70 kg person.

3. Commercially available combinations of local anesthetics and vasoconstrictors

Commonly available commercial combinations of local anesthetics and vasoconstrictors are listed in **Table 6.4**. It is important to have several different forms of the combinations available for the specific needs of the practice. It is also important to be comfortable with the combinations chosen so as not to exceed the maximal one-time dose administration.

TABLE 6.4 Commonly available forms of local anesthetic and vasoconstrictor combination

Generic	Brand name	Available forms
Lidocaine	Xylocaine	1% with 1:100,000 epinephrine 2% with 1:100,000 epinephrine 2% with 1:200,000 epinephrine 2% with 1:50,000 epinephrine
Articaine	Septocaine	4% with 1:100,000 epinephrine 4% with 1:200,000 epinephrine
Mepivacaine	Carbocaine	2% with 1:20,000 levonordefrin 3% without levonordefrin (plain)
Prilocaine	Citanest	3% without epinephrine (plain) 4% without epinephrine (plain) 4% with 1:200,000 epinephrine
Bupivacaine	Marcaine	0.25%, 0.5%, 0.75% with 1:200,000 epinephrine

4. Limitation of vasoconstrictors in patients with cardiovascular diseases

This is one of the most discussed issues in the use of local anesthetics with vasoconstrictors. Even judicious use of vasoconstrictors can result in the elevation of serum epinephrine with resultant elevation of blood pressure and/or arrhythmia.

It is clear that limitation to 2 carpules of 1:100,000 or epinephrine or 1:20,000 of levonordefrin or 4 carpules of 1:200,000 of epinephrine is generally safe for the hypertensive or cardiac patient **(Table 6.5)**. This can result in change in treatment plan and breaking up long procedures into several phases.

TABLE 6.5 Maximal one-time dose of vasoconstrictor in patients with cardiac contraindications*

Epinephrine 1:50,000	AVOID
Epinephrine 1:100,000	2 carpules
Epinephrine 1:200,000	4 carpules
Levonordefrin 1:20,000	2 carpules

*Estimated for a 70 kg person.

Being comfortable with the use of a selected number of local anesthetics, optimizing injection techniques and understanding the maximal one-time dose of local anesthetics and vasoconstrictor are important for the safety and comfort of the patient.

7 ANTIBIOTIC PREMEDICATION FOR PATIENTS WITH VALVULAR AND CARDIAC INDICATIONS

INTRODUCTION

Many dental procedures are known to result in transient bacteremia. The degree of bacteremia is in general low and normally does not present as a health risk. However, in certain susceptible patients, transient bacteremia can result in serious complications. It is therefore important to identify the susceptibility of the patients.

In general, antibiotic premedication has been advocated for patients with cardiac valvular disorders and intracardiac devices and in patients with prosthetic joints.

We will address premedications for patients with transplants (Chapters 25 and 28) and non-valvular indications (Chapter 8) in separate chapters.

1. Medical evaluation of patients with valvular disorder or intracardiac devices

Current guidelines have been updated to include a number of interventions and devices now employed for patients with cardiac conditions (Table 7.1).

Valvular pathology can now be addressed not only with prosthetic cardiac valves and homografts (usually bovine grafts) addressed via open-heart surgery, transcatheter procedures are often preferred in the appropriate candidate:

- Transcatheter aortic valve replacements are now common.
- Similarly, mitral valve clips can be placed via transcatheter interventions in patients with significant mitral regurgitations.
- Mitral regurgitation can also be repaired with annuloplasty rings and chords.

While these procedures are less invasive than traditional open-heart surgery, all of these devices are foreign materials in the blood stream and can be seeded by transient bacteremia. They all therefore require antibiotic premedication prior to dental procedures.

Some of the other indications for antibiotic premedication have not changed:

- Patients with previous bouts of infective endocarditis require premedication.
- Patients with certain congenital heart disease require premedication:
    - Unrepaired cyanotic CHD
    - First 6 months after congenital heart defect repair
    - Palliative shunts and conduits
    - Repaired CHD with residual defects at the site or adjacent to the site of a prosthetic device
- Cardiac transplant patients with valvular regurgitation require premedication.

Since the dental professionals may not be well versed with the forever evolving innovations in cardiac interventions, it is prudent to consult the patient's cardiologist if there are ambiguities.

TABLE 7.1 Need for premedication in patients with cardiac indications

Coverage needed only for patients with:
Prosthetic cardiac valve, including transcatheter-implanted prostheses and homografts
Prosthetic material used for cardiac valve repair, such as annuloplasty rings and chords
Previous bouts of infective endocarditis
Certain congenital heart diseases: ▪ Unrepaired cyanotic CHD ▪ First 6 months after congenital heart defect repair ▪ Palliative shunts and conduits
Repaired CHD with residual defects at the site or adjacent to the site of a prosthetic device
Cardiac transplant recipients with valve regurgitation

Equally importantly, it should be stressed that patients with coronary stents, pacemakers and defibrillators do not require antibiotic premedication.
For patients needing antibiotic premedication **(Table 7.2)**, amoxicillin 2 g given 30 to 60 minutes prior to dental interventions.
For patients with penicillin allergy, the current recommendation is to use Cephalexin 2 g 30 to 60 minutes prior to dental interventions. Since there is a likelihood of cross-reactivity between penicillin and Cephalexin, Cephalexin should not be used in patients with a history of anaphylaxis, urticaria or angioedema to penicillin or ampicillin. Clarithromycin or azithromycin can also be used. Clindamycin is generally to be avoided because of concerns of side effects.

TABLE 7.2 Antibiotic regimens used for premedications

No penicillin allergy	Penicillin allergy
Amoxicillin 2 g	Cephalexin* 2 g
	Clarithromycin or azithromycin 500 mg
Ampicillin 2 g IM or IV Ceftriaxone or Cefazolin 1 g IM or IV for patients not able to take medications orally	Ceftriaxone or Cefazolin 1 g IM or IV for patients not able to take medications orally
All medications should be given 30–60 minutes before procedure	

*Should not be used in patients with history of anaphylaxis, urticaria or angioedema to penicillin or ampicillin.

2. Dental procedures necessitating antibiotic premedication

All dental procedures that involve manipulation of gingival tissue or the periapical region of teeth or perforation of the oral mucosa necessitate antibiotic premedication in the susceptible patient **(Table 7.3)**.

Even minor procedures would necessitate premedication including biopsies, suture removals and placement of orthodontic bands.

TABLE 7.3 Types of dental procedures necessitating antibiotic premedication in the susceptible patient

All dental procedures that involve manipulation of gingival tissue or the periapical region of teeth or perforation of the oral mucosa including:
Biopsy
Suture removal
Placement of orthodontic band

It is clear that antibiotic premedication is now limited to very specific and a small subgroup of patients deemed to be at high risk. There is also an effort to limit the use of clindamycin in patients with penicillin allergy, with the recommendation of using cephalexin. It is prudent to consult the cardiologist if there is any ambiguity about the need for premedication.

8 ANTIBIOTIC PREMEDICATION FOR THE PATIENT WITH NON-VALVULAR INDICATIONS

INTRODUCTION

With the evolution of a myriad of medical devices, concerns have been raised about the need for premedication for dental procedures for these devices.

Bacteremia occurs with a large variety of dental interventions (Table 8.1), and considerations for premedication prior to dental procedures should be carefully considered for each individual case.

Unlike premedication of valvular heart disease, there are few guidelines for many of these devices. In many instances, the choice of premedication is left to the physician and patient. It is therefore important to have some general principles guiding these decisions and to have consultation with the relevant clinicians in order to provide optimal care to the patient.

An over-riding principle is the fact that when the device is exposed, antibiotic premedication is reasonable. Once the device is endothelialized, premedication is generally no longer necessary.

TABLE 8.1 Types of dental procedures associated with bacteremia

All dental procedures that involve manipulation of gingival tissue or the periapical region of teeth or perforation of the oral mucosa
Biopsy
Suture removal
Placement of orthodontic band

1. Vascular grafts

Vascular grafts are placed to replaced damaged vessels throughout the body and considerations for antibiotic premedication should be made in conjunction with the appropriate clinicians.

- **Coronary artery bypass grafts**
  Elective dental procedures are not recommended for the first 6 months following coronary artery bypass surgery. Beyond the first 6 months, the grafts are generally endothelialized and **antibiotic premedication is not necessary**.

- **Aortic grafts**
  It is reasonable to consider antibiotic premedication for the 6 months following graft placement. Beyond the first 6 months, the grafts are generally endothelialized and **antibiotic premedication is not necessary**.

- **Peripheral vascular grafts**
  It is reasonable to consider antibiotic premedication for the 6 months following graft placement. Beyond the first 6 months, the grafts are generally endothelialized and **antibiotic premedication is not necessary**.

2. Intracardiac devices

An increasing number of intracardiac devices are placed via percutaneous approach to aid with a variety of cardiac functions. It is important to realize that while the majority of these devices do not require antibiotic premedication, some devices have residual foreign materials or sutures that necessitate premedication.

- **Stents**
  Bare-metal stents and drug-eluting stents are placed for coronary artery stenoses or occlusions and **do not require antibiotic premedication**. There have been no reports of stents getting infected via hematogenous seeding.

- **Pacemakers**
  Pacemakers are placed in patients with conduction system disease and pacemaker wires **do not require antibiotic premedication**.

- **Defibrillators**
  Implantable cardioverter defibrillators and cardiac resynchronization therapy defibrillators are placed in patients susceptible to lethal arrhythmias such as ventricular fibrillation and ventricular tachycardia. Patients with congestive heart failure and severely compromised ejection fractions are prone to lethal arrhythmias and often have these devices in place.
  Defibrillators **do not require antibiotic premedication**.

- **Implanted cardiac loop recorder**
  Cardiac loop recorder may be implanted to allow for long-term monitoring of rhythm abnormalities. These **do not require antibiotic premedication**.

- **Transcatheter aortic valve replacement**
  Increasingly, aortic valves are replaced with a transcatheter approach. Since a mechanical valve has been placed, these patients **require life-long antibiotic premedication** for dental procedures.

- **Mitral valvuloplasty**
  For patients with mitral valve regurgitation, a mitral ring with mitral valvuloplasty is another minimally invasive procedure that can improve valvular competency. These patients **require life-long antibiotic premedication** for dental procedures.

- **WATCHMAN™ device**
  The major concern in patients with atrial fibrillation is the formation of clots in the left atrial appendage that can result in embolic events. Patients with atrial fibrillation are generally on anticoagulants. In patients with contraindication to anticoagulation, a WATCHMAN™ device, which allows for obliteration of the atrial appendage, is sometimes deployed. The device endothelializes within a short period of time. It is reasonable to premedicate only for the 6 months following the placement of the WATCHMAN™ device and not thereafter.

It is clear that many other devices will be available, but the need for premedication can be delineated by whether the devices are endothelialized. In instances where there are exposed grafts, mechanical surfaces or sutures, antibiotic premedication should be considered. In instances where the device is endothelialized, premedications are generally not necessary.
It is important to connect with the appropriate clinicians prior to elective dental interventions to coordinate the optimal management of the patient.

3. Dialysis accesses, hemodialysis and peritoneal dialysis

Patients with end stage renal disease are generally on hemodialysis where their blood is cleansed by a dialysis machine three to five times a week. A small percentage of patients are on peritoneal dialysis, where a catheter is surgically placed into the peritoneal cavity and the patient is on continuous exchanges. Infection of the accesses and the peritoneal space are constant concerns and antibiotic premedication is often considered prior to dental procedures. All decisions should be made in conjunction with the responsible nephrologist.

- **Arteriovenous fistula**
  The majority of patients on dialysis have arteriovenous conduits created in the antecubital or brachial space. These fistulae are accessed three times a week with large bore needles to facilitate dialysis.
  These are native vessels and **antibiotic premedication is generally not recommended**.

- **Arteriovenous graft**
  Arteriovenous grafts are used in a small proportion of dialysis patients in instances when the native vessel would not support an arteriovenous fistula. These are generally made of synthetic materials. Although the surface of the grafts does endothelialized, the fact that the access is repeatedly punctured would lead one to **recommend antibiotic premedication** for dental procedures.

- **Indwelling internal jugular catheters**
  In some patients, a double lumen tunneled catheter is placed in the internal jugular vein for dialysis, usually prior to placement of more permanent accesses. These are extremely prone to infection and **antibiotic premedication is generally recommended**.

- **Peritoneal dialysis catheters**
  Patients on peritoneal dialysis have an indwelling catheter in the peritoneal cavity and are susceptible to peritonitis. These are extremely prone to infection, and **antibiotic premedication is generally recommended**.

4. Intravascular ports and catheters

When repeated access to the patient's veins is necessary, ports and Hickman catheters may be placed. These are susceptible to infection, and considerations should be made for antibiotic premedication prior to dental procedures.

- **Ports**
  Ports are placed in patients who need reliable and reported venous access for infusion and for blood draw. Patients with cancer would have ports placed for chemotherapy. Patients with ports are at increased risk of infection due to the presence of a foreign substance and due to their underlying medical conditions. It is reasonable to **consider antibiotic premedication** prior to dental interventions.

- **Hickman catheter**
  Hickman catheter is a central venous catheter usually used in patients with cancer or other serious medical conditions. The catheters are susceptible to infection, and it is reasonable to **consider antibiotic premedication** prior to dental procedures

Because patients with ports and Hickman catheters are generally complicated patients with compromised immune systems, it is important to coordinate antibiotic premedication with the appropriate clinicians.

5. Intraventricular shunts

Intraventricular shunts are placed to decompress hydrocephalus. Two types of shunts are commonly employed and there are actual guidelines for antibiotic premedication use in these patients.

- **Ventriculo-atrial shunt**
  Antibiotic premedication is generally not necessary.

- **Ventriculo-peritoneal shunt**
  Antibiotic premedication **is generally recommended**.

6. Antibiotic premedication regimen

In general, standard premedication regimen would be appropriate.
If antibiotic premedication is deemed necessary, amoxicillin 2 g should be given an hour before planned procedure to patients without penicillin allergy (Table 8.2).
For patients with penicillin allergy, cephalexin 2 g should be given an hour before planned procedure. Cephalexin should not be used in patients with history of anaphylaxis, urticaria or angioedema to penicillin or ampicillin (Table 8.2).

TABLE 8.2 Antibiotics premedication regimen

Premedication given one hour before procedure	
No penicillin allergy	**Penicillin allergy**
Amoxicillin 2 g	Cephalexin 2 g Should not be used in patients with history of anaphylaxis, urticaria or angioedema to penicillin or ampicillin
	Azithromycin 500 mg

Patients with grafts and devices have special dental needs. It is important to attend to the oral health aggressively to minimize oral infection. The patient should be instructed on oral hygiene and home care to optimize oral health. These patients would benefit from frequent recalls after the first 6 months of transplant.
Because these patients are complicated, it is important to coordinate antibiotic premedication with the appropriate clinician.

9 ANTIBIOTIC PREMEDICATION FOR DENTAL PROCEDURES IN PATIENTS WITH PROSTHETIC JOINTS

INTRODUCTION

Many dental procedures are known to result in transient bacteremia. The degree of bacteremia is in general low and normally does not present as a health risk. However, in certain susceptible patients, transient bacteremia can result in serious complications. It is therefore important to identify the susceptibility of the patients.

Patients with prosthetic joints have very low likelihood of developing prosthetic joint infection as the result of bacteremia from dental procedures. **Premedication is therefore to be avoided except in a small group of patients deemed to be at high risk.**

1. Patients with prosthetic joints

The prosthetic joints under consideration are generally the weight bearing joints, hips and knees and do not include pins and plates.

Even with these joints, prosthetic joint infection as a result of dental procedures is an exceedingly rare event. In general, premedication is deemed not necessary.

Most prosthetic joint infection is caused by staphylococcal species.

Patients at potential risk (Table 9.1) are either heavily immunosuppressed or have diabetes under poor control. Although these patients have been considered as patients at risk and require premedication, there is a paucity of evidence supporting need for premedication even in these patients.

TABLE 9.1 Patients at potential risk for joint infection*

Immunocompromised status
Stage 3 AIDS (CD4 less than 200)
Cancer patients on immunosuppression
Cancer patients with fever/neutropenia
Rheumatoid arthritis on biologic or prednisone
Solid organ transplant on immunosuppression
Inherited diseases of immunodeficiency
Bone marrow transplant (pre and 100 days post)
Poor glycemic control

*AAOS Appropriate Use Criteria recommendation 2017

Since staphylococcal species is the most common organism in prosthetic joint infection, cephalosporin 2 g given orally should be the drug of choice **(Table 9.2).** In patients with Penicillin allergy with a history of anaphylaxis, urticaria or angioedema, clindamycin 600 mg should be considered.

If premedication is indeed deemed necessary, the prescription should be written by the orthopedic surgeon.

All medications should be given 60 minutes before procedure.

TABLE 9.2 Antibiotic prophylaxis for patients with prosthetic joints

No penicillin allergy	**Penicillin allergy**
Cephalexin 2 g preferred because of the excellent anti-staphylococcal coverage Amoxicillin 2 g	Cephalexin* 2 g
	Clindamycin 600 mg
All medications should be given 60 minutes before procedure	
If prophylaxis is deemed necessary, the prescription should be written by the orthopedic surgeon	

*Should not be used in patients with history of anaphylaxis, urticaria or angioedema to penicillin or ampicillin

2. Dental procedures necessitating antibiotic premedication

All dental procedures that involve manipulation of gingival tissue or the periapical region of teeth or perforation of the oral mucosa necessitate antibiotic premedication in the susceptible patient **(Table 9.3).**

Even minor procedures would necessitate premedication including biopsies, suture removals and placement of orthodontic bands.

TABLE 9.3 Types of dental procedures necessitating antibiotic premedication in the susceptible patient

All dental procedures that involve manipulation of gingival tissue or the periapical region of teeth or perforation of the oral mucosa including:
Biopsy
Suture removal
Placement of orthodontic band

In essence, there is little evidence that infection of the prosthetic joint can result from dental procedures. Since much of the decision is based upon clinical grounds of the patient's susceptibility and the type of prosthesis in place, it would be prudent for the orthopedic surgeon to decide upon need of premedication and to write the antibiotic prescription if premedication is deemed necessary.

10 ANTIBIOTICS IN MANAGEMENT OF PATIENTS WITH ACUTE DENTAL PAIN AND SWELLING

INTRODUCTION

One of the most common emergency presentations to the dental office is that of acute dental pain and swelling secondary to localized infection in the oral cavity in an immunocompetent patient. The guiding principles in management of these patients include:

- Identification of the extent of infection.
- Use of definitive conservative dental treatment should be prioritized. Being able to decompress the infected space is the key to successful management of patients with acute dental pain and swelling.
- Need for antibiotics is in large part predicated by the ability to perform definitive conservative management.
- Minimization of the use of antibiotics since they are of negligible benefit and are of significant harm, both to the patient and to the contribution to drug-resistant infections.
- Minimization of the use of clindamycin.

1. Extent of infection

The extent of infection **(Figure 10.1)** dictates the need for antibiotics in the patient presenting with acute pain and swelling. The extent of infection can be gauged by the clinical presentation: acute pain versus acute pain and swelling. More severe infection can be associated with systemic symptoms such as fever and lymphadenopathy.

- **Acute pain**
  - **Dental caries (Figure 10.1A)**
    All dental infections start with bacteria invading dental caries.
  - **Symptomatic irreversible pulpitis (Figure 10.1B)**
    When the infection invades the pulp, the patient will present with acute pain.
  - **Symptomatic apical periodontitis (Figure 10.1C)**
    As the infection progresses, apical periodontitis can occur. The patient will present with acute pain.

- **Acute pain and swelling**
  - **Pulp necrosis (Figure 10.1D)**
    As the infection progresses, the patient will develop pain and swelling as the pulp becomes necrosed. The patient will present with pain and swelling.
  - **Localized apical abscess (Figure 10.1E)**
    The patient will present with pain and swelling.

- **Systemic involvement**
  The patient may present with fever or evidence of extension of the infection to involve lymph nodes. Presence of systemic involvement mandates antibiotic treatment.

FIGURE 10.1 Stages of odontogenic infections

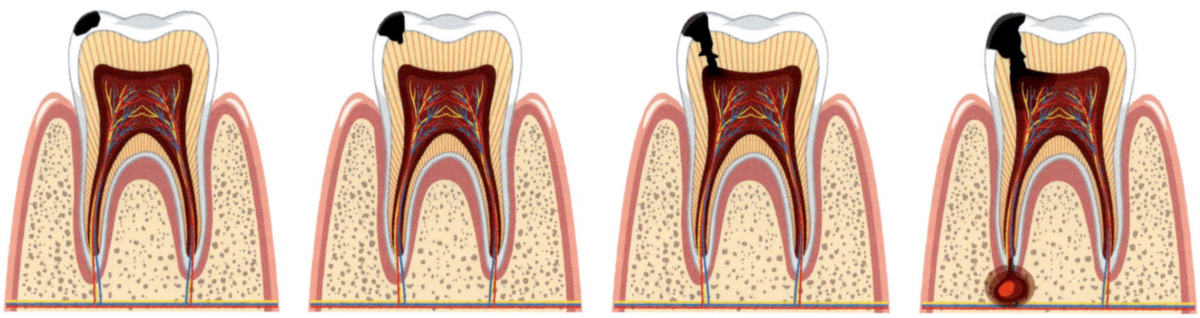

10.1A Dental caries

10.1B Symptomatic irreversible pulpitis

10.1C Symptomatic apical periodontitis

10.1D Pulpal necrosis

10.1E Localized apical abscess

2. Availability of definitive conservative dental treatment

Dental pain and swelling are best managed with decompression of the infected space. Definitive conservative dental treatments should always be prioritized. Use of antibiotics in the management of inadequately decompressed infected space is generally not desirable.

The different definitive conservative dental treatment options are listed in **Table 10.1**. These are all procedures designed to unroof the infected space. Without decompression of the infected space, antibiotics alone are generally ineffective. With the decompression, antibiotic therapy may not be necessary.

TABLE 10.1 Definitive conservative dental treatment

Pulpotomy
Pulpectomy
Non-surgical root canal treatment
Incision and drainage

3. Need for antibiotics

The need for antibiotics is predicated on both the extent of infection and the availability of definitive conservative dental treatment.

- **Acute pain (symptomatic irreversible pulpitis or symptomatic apical periodontitis)**
  When a patient presents with acute pain only, antibiotics should not be prescribed. They are of negligible benefit in this instance.

- **Acute pain and swelling (pulp necrosis with or without localized apical abscess)**
  Definitive conservative dental treatment should be prioritized. Antibiotics are not necessary if definitive conservative dental treatments can be carried out.
  However, if definitive conservative dental treatments are not immediately available, the patient may benefit from a short course of antibiotics until decompressive treatments can be carried out, particularly if there is evidence of localized apical abscess. In instances where only pulpal necrosis is present clinically, it is reasonable to withhold antibiotics unless there is clinical progression of symptoms.

- **Systemic involvement**
  Antibiotics are necessary in all patients with clinical evidence of systemic involvement.

4. Antibiotic regimen for management of patient with acute dental pain and swelling

In general, management of patients without penicillin allergy should involve either amoxicillin or penicillin VK for 3-7 days.

If anaerobic coverage is deemed necessary, the antibiotic should be switched to Augmentin **(Table 10.2)**.

In patients with penicillin allergy, cephalexin should be used since there is a significant shift to minimizing the use of clindamycin. Cephalexin should not be used in patients with history of anaphylaxis, urticaria or angioedema to penicillin or ampicillin.

Azithromycin, given in either a 3-day or a 5-day course can also be used in penicillin allergic patients **(Table 10.2)**.

In instances where anaerobic coverage is needed, metronidazole can be added onto the existing antibiotic regimen. It is important to caution patients on metronidazole not to consume alcohol since metronidazole has an Antabuse effect.

TABLE 10.2 Antibiotics for management of patients with acute pain and swelling

Antibiotics if clinically indicated	
No penicillin allergy	**Penicillin allergy**
Amoxicillin 500 mg TID or Amoxicillin 875 mg BID for 3-7 days	Cephalexin* 500 mg QID
Penicillin VK 500 mg TID for 3-7 days	Azithromycin 500 mg Day 1 250 mg Days 2-5 or Azithromycin 500 mg QD for 3 days
Switch to Augmentin 500 mg TID or Augmentin 875 mg BID for 7 days	
Add metronidazole 500 mg TID for 7 days Caution not to consume alcohol (Antabuse effect)	

*Should not be used in patients with history of anaphylaxis, urticaria or angioedema to penicillin or ampicillin

These current guidelines prioritize the use of definitive conservative dental treatment to unroof the infection, thus minimizing the need for antibiotics. In instances where there are clinical signs of systemic involvement, antibiotics should be prescribed, with careful follow-up.

11 ANTIBIOTIC THERAPY FOR DENTAL IMPLANT PLACEMENT

INTRODUCTION

Most dental professionals prescribe antibiotics around the time of the dental implant placements. There are many different protocols with different antibiotic regimens proposed. The results of various trials have been variable, making concrete guidelines difficult to justify.

In general, it is important to limit the use of antibiotics whenever feasible. The need should be dependent upon the patient's medical condition, the presence of chronic infection and the procedure planned.

Antibiotics can be prescribed as a single dose premedication, a short course after the implant placement or both.

1. Rationale for using antibiotics

Dental implants can fail due to multiple reasons. However, infection is often an important concern. Antibiotic use is aimed at preventing or treating bacterial infections that may be present. Antibiotics can be prescribed as antibiotic premedication or as a short course of antibiotics following the implant. However, data showing actual improvement of implant success is currently spotty and there is little consensus around the proper use of antibiotics for dental implant placement.

In 2022, Spanish dental professionals arrived at a consensus opinion governing the use of antibiotics for healthy patients receiving dental implants. Considerations were made according to the procedures planned, the status of the bone and the presence of infection at the implant sites. These all play a role in the decision of the need for premedication and the need for subsequent course of antibiotics.

2. Simple implants in healthy patients

In healthy patients without anatomical constraints who need a simple implant, with or without bone regeneration procedures, the Spanish consensus recommend a single dose of premedication.

For patients without penicillin allergy, the recommended regimen is amoxicillin 2–3 g as a single dose one hour before the procedure **(Table 11.1).**

For patients allergic to penicillin, a single dose of azithromycin 500 mg given an hour before the procedure is recommended **(Table 11.1).**

TABLE 11.1 Antibiotics for simple implants in healthy patients

Premedication given one hour before procedure	
No penicillin allergy	**Penicillin allergy**
Amoxicillin 3 g	Azithromycin 500 mg

3. Immediate dental implants

Immediate dental implants may involve some degree of chronic infection of the tooth/teeth to be extracted. In addition to the single dose premedication, antibiotics are recommended to continue for 5–7 days following the procedure.

For patients without penicillin allergy, amoxicillin 875 mg BID or amoxicillin 500 mg TID should be given for 5–7 days after the procedure **(Table 11.2).**

For patients allergic to penicillin, azithromycin 250 mg QD should be given for 5–7 days after the procedure **(Table 11.2).**

TABLE 11.2 Antibiotics for immediate dental implants in healthy patients

Premedication given one hour before procedure	
No penicillin allergy	**Penicillin allergy**
Amoxicillin 3 g premed	Azithromycin 500 mg premed
Amoxicillin 875 mg BID or Amoxicillin 500 mg TID for 5 to 7 days thereafter	Azithromycin 250 mg QD for 5 to 7 days thereafter

4. Dental implants involving sinus lifts

In instances where sinus lifts (transcrestal and/or lateral window approach), broad spectrum antibiotics are recommended.

For patients without penicillin allergy, amoxicillin-clavulanic acid (Augmentin) 875 mg BID or 500 mg TID should be started for one day before the procedure and continued for 7 days following the procedure **(Table 11.3).**

For patients allergic to penicillin, ciprofloxacin 500 mg BID should be started one day before the procedure and continue for 7 days thereafter **(Table 11.3).**

TABLE 11.3 Antibiotics for dental implants involving sinus lifts

Premedication given one hour before procedure	
No penicillin allergy	**Penicillin allergy**
Augmentin 875 mg premed	Ciprofloxacin 500 mg premed
Augmentin 875 mg BID or Augmentin 500 mg TID for 7 days thereafter	Ciprofloxacin 500 mg BID for 7 days thereafter

5. Prosthetic phase

During the prosthetic phase of dental implant procedures, no preventive antibiotic therapy is recommended.

Proper use of antibiotics around the time of the dental implant procedure is still an evolving concept. Based upon the Spanish consensus, we currently have a framework of reference around which further studies can be conducted.

12 ANTIBIOTIC THERAPY FOR ODONTOGENIC INFECTIONS

INTRODUCTION

Antibiotics are frequently used in dentistry. However, concerns have been raised about excessive and inappropriate use. In general, antibiotic use should be limited and clindamycin use, in particular, should be curtailed. Guidelines for antibiotic use address immunocompetent patients. Antibiotic use should be much more liberal in immunocompromised hosts with infection.

In the management of odontogenic infections, it is important to differentiate between localized and spreading infections.

Spreading infections mandate prompt intervention and aggressive treatment with antibiotics.

In contrast, management of localized infection in immunocompetent patients is best accomplished by definitive conservative dental treatment **(Table 12.1).** With successful drainage of the infected space, antibiotics may not be necessary.

1. Localized versus spreading infection

The extent of the infection needs to be defined whenever antibiotic use is considered.

Localized infection generally presents with acute dental pain and swelling. Occasionally, localized infection may be detected on routine dental radiographs. Localized infection should be managed by definitive conservative dental treatment. Adequately drained, antibiotics may not be needed.

Spreading infection occurs when the infection has extended beyond the immediate confines of the tooth and the surrounding gingival tissues. Spreading infections are medically complicated. They should be addressed with conservative dental treatments and antibiotics. In many instances, spreading infections may require surgical drainage and intravenous antibiotics.

2. Definitive conservative dental treatment

In odontogenic infections, the key to management is the prompt deployment of definitive conservative dental treatment. The ability to open up the infected space is crucial to the success of treatment. Table 12.1 lists the procedures commonly used: pulpotomy, pulpectomy, root canal and incision and drainage should be deployed in the appropriate clinical situations. All of these procedures will unroof the infected space and will often obviate the need for antibiotics altogether.

TABLE 12.1 Definitive conservative dental treatment (DCDT)

Pulpotomy
Pulpectomy
Non-surgical root canal treatment
Incision and drainage

3. Management of localized infection

The need for antibiotics in the management of localized infection is dependent upon the clinical presentation and access to immediate definitive conservative dental treatment (Table 12.1).

The most common presentation of localized odontogenic infections is pain and swelling at the affected site in immunocompetent patients. Patients can present with acute pain or acute pain and swelling.

All odontogenic infections begin with dental caries (Figure 12.1A). Patients with acute pain may have symptomatic **irreversible pulpitis (SIP)** (Figure 12.1B) with or without **symptomatic apical periodontitis (SAP)** (Figure 12.1C).

Patients with acute pain and localized swelling may have **pulp necrosis (PN)** (Figure 12.1D) and **symptomatic apical periodontitis (SAP)** (Figure 12.1C) or **pulp necrosis (PN)** and **localized apical abscess (LAA)** (Figure 12.1E).

FIGURE 12.1 Stages of odontogenic infection

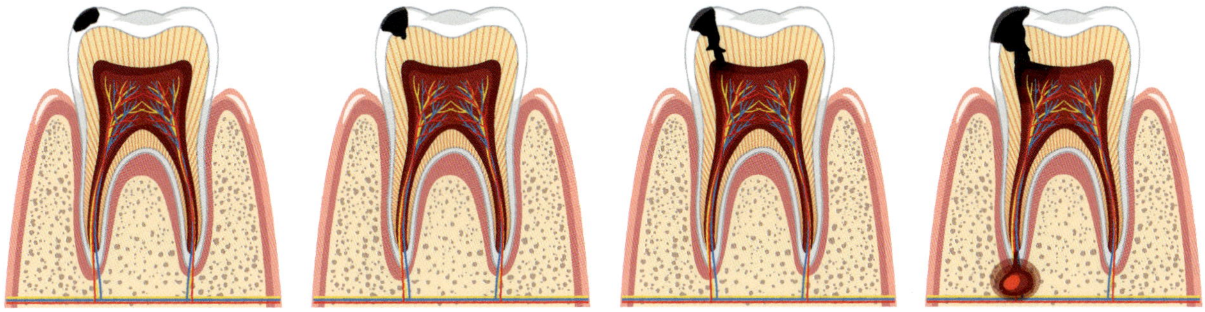

12.1A Dental caries	12.1B Symptomatic irreversible pulpitis 12.1C Symptomatic apical periodontitis	12.1D Pulpal necrosis	12.1E Localized apical abscess

In some instances, patients may actually have **systemic symptoms** of fevers and chills. These patients warrant antibiotic treatment.

In the management of localized odontogenic infections, the ability to access definitive conservative dental treatments **(Table 12.1)** is critical in controlling the infection and in minimizing the need for antibiotics.

If definitive conservative dental treatments can be promptly instituted, patients can generally manage without antibiotics **(Figure 12.2).** After treatment, patients with SIP, SAP, PN and LAA do not need antibiotics as adjunct to definitive conservative dental treatments. Only patients with evidence of systemic involvement will need antibiotics.

FIGURE 12.2 Antibiotics in management of patient with acute dental pain and swelling when definitive conservative dental treatment is immediately available

LOCALIZED INFECTION in immunocompetent patient			Definitive conservative dental treatment immediately available
Patient presentation			
Acute pain	Symptomatic irreversible pulpitis (SIP) with or without symptomatic apical periodontitis (SAP)	➜	No antibiotics
Acute pain and swelling	Pulp necrosis (PN) and symptomatic apical periodontitis (SAP)	➜	No antibiotics as adjunct to DCDT
	Pulp necrosis (PN) and localized apical abscess (LAA)	➜	No antibiotics as adjunct to DCDT
With systemic involvement		➜	*Antibiotics*

If definitive conservative dental treatments cannot be immediately accessed, antibiotic need is predicated on the clinical presentation. Patients presenting with acute pain only (SIP with or without SAP) do not need antibiotics. Patients presenting with pain and swelling may have PN and SAP. The recommendation is to manage either without antibiotics or with delayed antibiotics, where the patient is given a prescription and told to not fill the prescription unless their symptoms worsen. This would minimize unnecessary use of antibiotics.

FIGURE 12.3 Antibiotics in management of patient with acute dental pain and swelling when definitive conservative dental treatment is not immediately available

LOCALIZED INFECTION in immunocompetent patient			Definitive conservative dental treatment NOT immediately available	Definitive conservative dental treatment immediately available
Patient presentation				
Acute pain	Symptomatic irreversible pulpitis (SIP) with or without symptomatic apical periodontitis (SAP)	➜	No antibiotics	No antibiotics
Acute pain and swelling	Pulp necrosis (PN) and symptomatic apical periodontitis (SAP)	➜	No antibiotics or delayed antibiotics	No antibiotics as adjunct to DCDT
	Pulp necrosis (PN) and localized apical abscess (LAA)	➜	Antibiotics	No antibiotics as adjunct to DCDT
With systemic involvement		➜	*Antibiotics*	

For patients needing antibiotic therapy **(Table 12.2)**, amoxicillin 500 mg three times a day or amoxicillin 875 mg twice a day should be given for 3–7 days. The duration should be governed clinically by the severity of the infection.

For patients with penicillin allergy, the current recommendation is to use cephalexin **(Table 12.2)** in an attempt to minimize use of clindamycin. Since there is a likelihood of cross-reactivity between penicillin and cephalexin, cephalexin should not be used in patients with a history of anaphylaxis, urticaria or angioedema to penicillin or ampicillin. Cephalexin should be prescribed in 500 mg QID for 3–7 days. The duration is again governed by the severity of the infection.

Clarithromycin or azithromycin can also be used.

Clindamycin is generally to be avoided because of concerns over *C. difficile* colitis. It can be used when clinically indicated, particularly if anaerobic infection is suspected. The prescriber needs to inform the patient about this potential complication and to instruct the patient to stop the antibiotics if diarrhea occurs. Patients should be instructed to stop the antibiotic and contact the dental professional if diarrhea occurs. Stopping the antibiotic promptly often would allow the bowel flora to return to equilibrium within 24 hours. However, if the diarrhea persists beyond 24 hours, the patient will need medical attention for management of presumed *C. difficile* colitis.

Metronidazole is an important "add-on" antibiotic for refractory anaerobic infections. It is prescribed in 500 mg TID for 7 days. It is important to instruct the patient not to take alcohol during the duration of metronidazole use since the drug has a strong Antabuse effect.

TABLE 12.2 Antibiotics for odontogenic infections

Antibiotics if clinically indicated	
No penicillin allergy	**Penicillin allergy**
Amoxicillin 500 mg TID (or 875 mg BID) for 3-7 days	Cephalexin* 500 QID for 3-7 days
Penicillin VK 500 mg QID for 3-7 days	Azithromycin Z-Pak #1 as directed or Tri-Pak #1 as directed
	Clindamycin 300 mg QID for 3-7 days Clindamycin should be used judiciously
Add metronidazole (Flagyl) 500 mg TID for 7 days if necessary Caution not to consume alcohol (Antabuse effect) or	
Switch to Augmentin 500 mg TID (or 875 mg BID) for 7 days	

*Patient did not have hives, angioedema or anaphylaxis with penicillin

4. Management of spreading infection

Spreading infection occurs when the infection has reached beyond the immediate gingival tissue. Oral organisms in these spaces can pose significant morbidity. Spreading infection needs to be addressed immediately by definitive conservative dental intervention and aggressive use of antibiotics.

Spreading infections (Table 12.3) can present as cellulitis, fistulous tract to the face or jaw or involvement of the sinus space. After definitive conservative dental treatment, these infections can be managed with aggressive oral antibiotics (Table 12.4), with attention to anaerobic coverage.

In patients without penicillin allergy, amoxicillin-clavulonic acid (Augmentin) 500 mg TID or 875 mg BID is given for 7 days. Metronidazole 500 mg TID for 7 days can be added if additional anaerobic coverage is desired.

In patients with penicillin allergy, clindamycin 300 mg TID for 7 days may be appropriate since extended anaerobic coverage is desired. Patients should be warned to stop the

antibiotic and contact the dental professional if diarrhea occurs. Stopping the antibiotic promptly often would allow the bowel flora to return to equilibrium. However, if the diarrhea persists beyond 24 hours, the patient will need medical attention for the management of presumed *C. difficile* colitis.
Cephalexin can be used, but it has less anaerobic coverage than clindamycin.
Metronidazole can be added on in instances when anaerobic coverage is necessary.
Some spreading infections become serious medical concerns. It is still critical to drain the infected sites, but further interventions and intravenous antibiotics may be necessary.
Spreading infections can involve the retropharyngeal space. This is a medical emergency and would often involve surgical drainage and intravenous antibiotics. In severe instances, spreading infections can present with metastatic abscesses to the lungs and the brain. These would be managed with surgical or percutaneous drainage procedure and prolonged courses of intravenous antibiotics.

TABLE 12.3 Types of spreading infections

Cellulitis
Facial fistulization
Sinusitis
Retropharyngeal space
Brain abscess
Distant seeding

TABLE 12.4 Treatment of spreading infection

No penicillin allergy	**Penicillin allergy**
	Clindamycin 300 mg TID for 7 days
Augmentin 500 TID (or 875 mg BID) for 7 days	Cephalexin* 500 QID for 7 days
Add metronidazole (Flagyl) 500 mg TID if necessary Caution patient not to drink alcohol (Antabuse effect)	

* Penicillin allergy did not involve hives, angioedema or anaphylaxis

Spreading infections can present with metastatic seeding of oral organism forming abscesses in the lungs or brain. These are medical emergencies necessitating surgical or percutaneous drainage and prolonged courses of antibiotics. However, it is still critical to render definitive conservative dental treatment to drain the original site of infection.

13 THE MOST COMMONLY PRESCRIBED MEDICATIONS IN DENTISTRY FOR THE PEDIATRIC PATIENT

INTRODUCTION

The dental professional should be familiar with a number of medications they are likely to prescribe to their pediatric patients. While it is difficult to anticipate all of the drugs that might be appropriate for any given patient, the following limited list of medications would be appropriate in the majority of the instances.

1. Antibiotics

Antibiotics are commonly prescribed in dentistry. The proper deployment of antibiotics for premedication and for treatment of odontogenic infections is detailed in Chapters 7–11 and 12.

While there are unique circumstances where special antibiotics may be appropriate, the four most commonly prescribed antibiotics in **Table 13.1** would represent >90% of the clinical situations where antibiotics are prescribed for the pediatric patient.

Because of the unique composition of the oral flora, penicillin-based antibiotics remain one of the most frequently prescribed medication in dental practices. Although penicillin VK is still prescribed, its dosing schedule (QID) results in more common use of amoxicillin and amoxicillin-clavulonic acid (BID or TID).

Both amoxicillin and amoxicillin-clavulonic acid can be dosed in a BID dosing, which is more convenient for the patient resulting in higher compliance. Amoxicillin-clavulonic acid is generally prescribed in instances where there is concern over anaerobic infection. Clindamycin is to be avoided in children.

Cephalexin is now increasingly proposed for patients with a history of penicillin allergic reactions. However, there is a small chance of cross-reactivity (5–29%) with penicillin with immediate reaction. It should therefore not be prescribed for patients whose penicillin allergy involved angioedema, urticaria or anaphylaxis. It is prescribed as 25 to 50 mg/kg/day in divided TID doses.

Azithromycin is a good alternative for patients with penicillin allergy, but it does not have as good an anaerobic coverage. It is prescribed as 12 mg/kg/day in QD dosing.

Although clarithromycin is a macrolide similar to azithromycin, its metabolism by CYP3A4 leads to drug-drug interaction not seen with azithromycin. In general, one should use azithromycin whenever a macrolide is considered.

TABLE 13.1 Antibiotics commonly prescribed to the pediatric patient

Amoxicillin	40 mg/kg/day in divided BID or TID doses
Amoxicillin-clavulonic acid	45 mg/kg/day in divided BID or TID doses
Azithromycin	12 mg/kg/day QD for 5 days
Cephalexin	25 to 50 mg/kg/day in divided TID doses

2. Analgesics in the pediatric patient

In general, acetaminophen should be the foundation for pain control in the pediatric patient and non-steroidal anti-inflammatory drugs can be added to synergize its efficacy. The proper use of analgesics and anti-inflammatory drugs is detailed in Chapter 4.

For mild pain, acetaminophen is the most logical analgesic to use. Acetaminophen can be administered in doses of 10-15 mg/kg/dose every 4-6 hours.

In instances where additional analgesia is desired, non-steroidal anti-inflammatory drugs can be added to acetaminophen **(Table 13.2).**

Non-steroidal anti-inflammatory drugs can cause gastrointestinal irritation. They are contraindicated in patients with pre-existing renal insufficiency since it can precipitate acute kidney injury. The most commonly prescribed non-steroidal anti-inflammatory drugs in the pediatric patient are ibuprofen and naproxen. Ibuprofen is administered in 4-10 mg/kg/dose every 5-8 hours. Naproxen is administered in 10 mg/kg/day in divided BID dosing.

TABLE 13.2 Commonly prescribed analgesics and anti-inflammatory drugs in the pediatric patient

Acetaminophen	10-15 mg/kg/dose Q4-6 hour
Ibuprofen	4-10 mg/kg/dose Q6-8 hour
Naproxen	10 mg/kg/day in divided BID doses

3. Opioids in the pediatric patient

Opioid use in dentistry has drawn scrutiny, particularly in the pediatric patient (Table 13.3). It should be reserved for the rare instances where one cannot get adequate pain control at maximal doses of analgesics and anti-inflammatory drugs.

Acetaminophen should be added to the narcotic to optimize efficacy. Although commercially available combinations of acetaminophen and narcotics are commonly prescribed, one should get used to prescribing acetaminophen separately from the opioids. This would permit more careful titration of opioid use.

TABLE 13.3 Commonly prescribed narcotics in the pediatric patient

Oxycodone	2.5 mg every 8 hours
Demerol	1-1.5 mg/kg/dose Q3-4 hours
Codeine	1-1.5 mg/kg/day in divided Q6 hours doses

In general, one ought to be comfortable with the use of these limited number of medications, which should constitute 90% of medications prescribed to the pediatric patient.

14 MEDICATION-RELATED OSTEONECROSIS OF THE JAW

INTRODUCTION

Medication-related osteonecrosis of the jaw is a rare but debilitating disease. It is characterized by exposed and non-healing bone in the jaw with severe sequelae. Since over 70% of the cases of medication related osteonecrosis of the jaw are associated with dental procedures such as extractions and implant placement, it is important that dental professionals make the appropriate assessment of risks in every instance where medications the patients are on can be associated with this complication.

In general, medication-related osteonecrosis of the jaw is associated with anti-resorptive agents used primarily for osteoporosis or with anti-angiogenic agents used for chemotherapy. All patients with current or prior exposure to these agents ought to be identified, the risks should be stratified, and dental treatment should be adjusted according to the risk profile.

1. Anti-resorptives (bisphosphonates and RANK-L inhibitors)

Anti-resorptives inhibit osteoclastic activity in the bone and are clinically used to manage osteoporosis. In rare instances, anti-resorptives, generally in much higher doses, can be used to manage bone cancer, primary or metastatic.

- **Anti-resorptive: bisphosphonates in management of osteoporosis**
  Bone turns over continuously by a balance between osteoblasts which deposit new bone and osteoclasts which rid the old bone. As patients age, osteoblastic activity slows down, causing decrease in bone density, osteopenia, which progress to osteoporosis that renders the bone vulnerable to pathological fractures. Oral bisphosphonates are the mainstay of management of osteoporosis, and it is estimated that

globally 45 million prescriptions are written each year (Table 14.1). Bisphosphonates are imbedded into the bone and would impair osteoclastic activity by causing osteoclast death when they are ingested (Figure 14.1). Bone density is therefore better preserved and pathological fractures are minimized on bisphosphonate therapy. However, the bone structure is not of normal integrity since bone turnover has been compromised. These bones would heal poorly, hence contributing to osteonecrosis in the appropriate setting.

Osteonecrosis of the jaw has been described with all bisphosphonates used for management of osteoporosis, although the incidence is quite low (Table 14.1).

Once bisphosphonate is imbedded in the bone, it remains for up to a decade. It is therefore now more common to prescribe bisphosphonates for 4–5 years only. Other drugs are now available for management of osteoporosis.

- **Anti-resorptive: RANK-L inhibitors in management of osteoporosis**

  RANK-L inhibitors prevent the formation of osteoclasts from the precursors (Figure 14.2). Although the mechanism of decreasing osteoclastic activity is different, these inhibitors have also been shown to be associated with osteonecrosis of the jaw (Table 14.1). The incidence is also quite low when RANK-L inhibitors are used for management of osteoporosis.

TABLE 14.1 Anti-resorptives for osteoporosis associated with osteonecrosis of the jaw

Osteoporosis: Oral bisphosphonates
Alendronate (Fosamax, Fosamax Plus D)
Risedronate (Actonel)
Ibandronate (Boniva)
Etidronate (Didronel)
Very low risk Incidence 0.04–0.3%

Osteoporosis: IV bisphosphonates
Zoledronic acid (Reclast) ◆ usually administered every 12 months
Very low risk

Osteoporosis: RANK-L inhibitor
Denosumib (Prolia) ◆ usually administered every 6 months
Very low risk

FIGURE 14.1

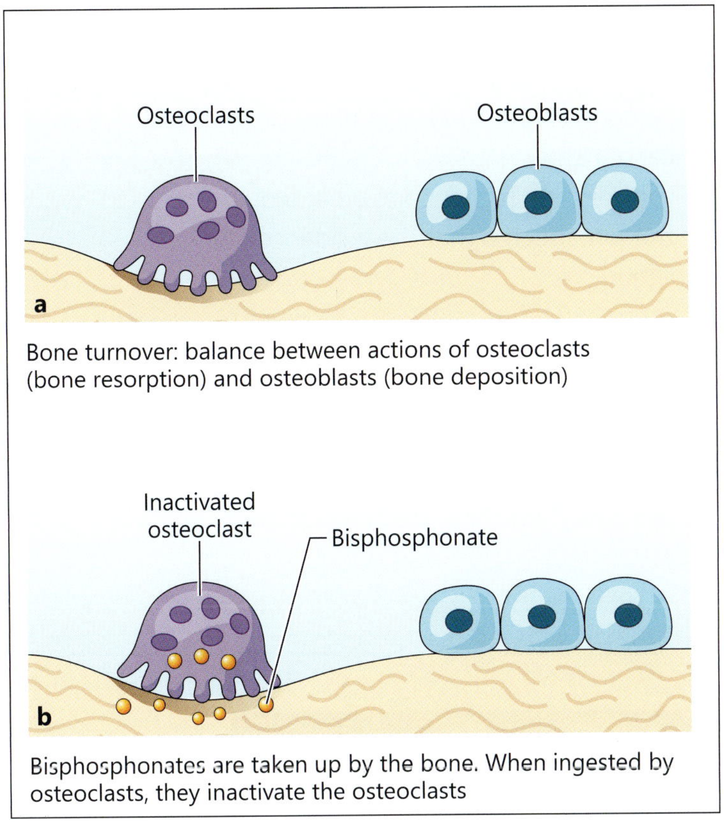

a Bone turnover: balance between actions of osteoclasts (bone resorption) and osteoblasts (bone deposition)

b Bisphosphonates are taken up by the bone. When ingested by osteoclasts, they inactivate the osteoclasts

FIGURE 14.2

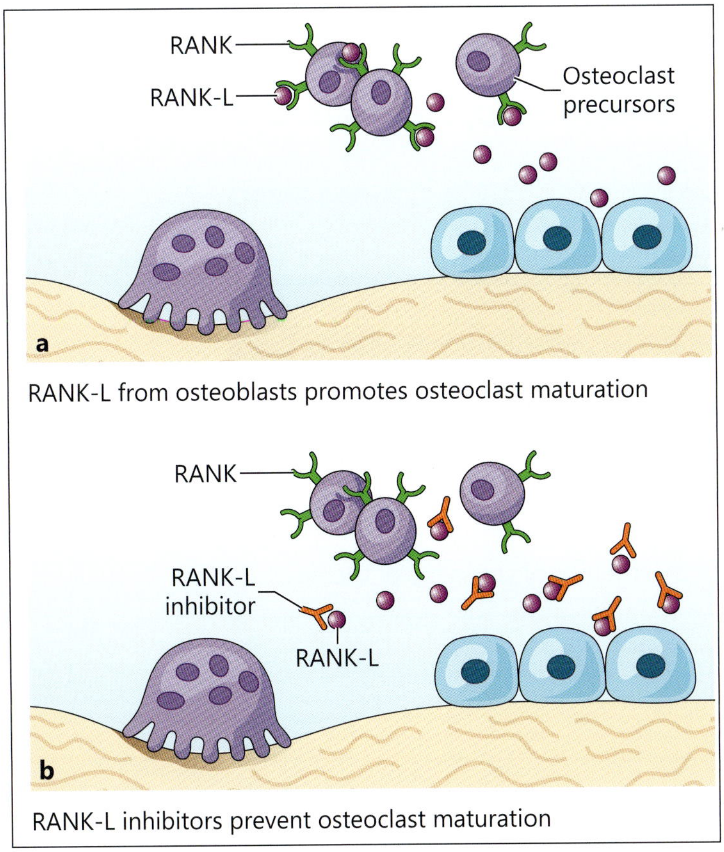

a RANK-L from osteoblasts promotes osteoclast maturation

b RANK-L inhibitors prevent osteoclast maturation

- **Anti-resorptive: bisphosphonates in management of bone cancers**

  Bisphosphonate is important in the management of primary bone cancer such as multiple myeloma or metastatic disease to the bone **(Table 14.2).** It is particularly helpful in the management of bone pain in cancer patients.

  In these instances, the doses prescribed are considerably higher than what would be prescribed for osteoporosis. It is therefore not unexpected that the incidence of osteonecrosis of the jaw is also considerably higher.

  It is therefore important to identify these patients and aggressively try to do aggressive preventive measures in these patients.

- **Anti-resorptive: RANK-L inhibitors in management of bone cancers**

  RANK-L inhibitors are occasionally used for bone cancer and metastatic cancer to the bone. The doses are considerably higher, and they have also been associated with osteonecrosis of the jaw **(Table 14.2).**

TABLE 14.2 Risks of development of osteonecrosis of the jaw with anti-resorptives in the management of cancer

Cancer patients: **IV bisphosphonates**
Zoledronic Acid (Zometa)
Pamidronate (Aredia)
Clodronate (Bonefos)
Significant risk **Incidence 0.8-6.7%**

Cancer patients: **RANK-L inhibitor**
Denosumab (Xgeva) ◆ for reducing skeletal related events in metastatic bone disease ◆ usually administered monthly ◆ do not bind to bone ◆ effect on bone remodeling diminished within 6 months of cessation of therapy
Significant risk

2. Anti-angiogenic treatment of patients with solid tumors

Anti-angiogenic agents are increasingly used for treatment of solid tumors. Solid tumors produce a vascular endothelial growth factor (VEGF) that promotes vascular growth and blood supply to the tumor. The identification of the VEGF permits the manufacturing of VEGF inhibitors, which will hamper tumor growth by interfering with its vascular supply. Tyrosine kinase inhibitors such as sunitinib and sorafenib and monoclonal antibodies to VEGF (bevacizumab) are now in clinical use. Unfortunately, these agents have been associated with osteonecrosis of the jaw, presumably because of interference of growth of new vasculature necessary for healing **(Table 14.3).**

Although all previous emphasis has been on identification of patients at risk receiving osteoporosis treatment, the increasing use of anti-angiogenic agents in chemotherapy is making it important not to overlook this patient population. The exact risk of these anti-angiogenic agents is still being assessed.

TABLE 14.3 Antiangiogenic agents associated with osteonecrosis of the jaw

Cancer patients: antiangiogenic agents
VEGF inhibitors
Tyrosine kinase inhibitors
◆ Sunitinib (Sutent)
◆ Sorafenib (Nexavar)
Monoclonal antibodies to VEGF
◆ Bevacizumab (Avastin)
Significant risk

3. Risk assessment of medication-related osteonecrosis of the jaw

By far the most important aspect of minimizing the risk of osteonecrosis is the prompt identification of patients at risk. Most dental professionals are quite accustomed to having questions in the patient questionnaire identifying those that have been exposed to bisphosphonates **(Table 14.4).** It is recommended that the questionnaire be worded to be able to identify patients that might be on anti-angiogenic agents as well **(Table 14.4).**

TABLE 14.4 Identification of patients potentially at risk for osteonecrosis of the jaw

Patients with osteoporosis
Have you ever been or are currently in treatment for osteoporosis?
Which agent(s) have been used?
How long were you or have you been in treatment?
Patients with cancer
Have you ever been or are currently in treatment for cancer?
Which agent(s) have been used?
How long were you or have you been in treatment?

Equally importantly, the procedure planned plays an important role in the assessment of risk of development of osteonecrosis of the jaw. In general, the more invasive the procedure is with respect to dental trauma, the higher the risk.
In general, patients in treatment for osteoporosis are at substantially lower risk than patients in treatment for cancer.

- **Risk assessment of patients on anti-resorptives for osteoporosis**

  In general, treatment with anti-resorptive for osteoporosis carries a very small risk of osteonecrosis of the jaw **(Table 14.5).** The risk increases with advancing age (greater than age 65) and duration of therapy (greater than 4 years). Presence of oral infection and pre-existing dental disease also increases risk.

  Other cited risk factors that may play a role include diabetes mellitus, steroid use, prior head and neck radiation. While there are reports of association with alcohol and tobacco use, these associations appear to play a minor role.

TABLE 14.5 Risk assessment of patients on oral or intravenous bisphosphonates for treatment of osteoporosis

Risk factors	Supporting evidence
Duration of therapy >4 years	+
Age >65	+
Oral infection	+
Pre-existing dental disease	+
Diabetes mellitus	+/-
Steroid use	+/-
Head and neck radiation	+
Alcohol use	+/-
Tobacco use	+/-
Anatomical anomalies	+/-

- **Risk assessment of patients on anti-resorptives for cancer**

High dose intravenous bisphosphonates used in treatment of cancer poses a very high risk for development of osteonecrosis of the jaw. Risks increase with duration of therapy. In one study, 12.5% of patients developed osteonecrosis of the jaw after 36 months of therapy with IV zoledronic acid (Zometa).
The risk is further compounded if the patient is also on anti-resorptive for osteoporosis.

- **Risk assessment of patients on anti-angiogenic agents for solid tumors**

While the exact risk of development of osteonecrosis of the jaw for each anti-angiogenic agent used for treatment of solid tumors has not been defined, it appears that it is probably as high as that of high dose anti-resorptive. The risk is accentuated if the patient is also taking an anti-resorptive. The risk increases with duration on anti-angiogenic agents.

4. Minimizing risks in patients on anti-resorptives

Correct identification of susceptive patients is the most important factor in the minimization of risk of development of osteonecrosis of the jaw.

- **Patients at low risk**

  Patients below the age of 65 who have been on anti-resorptives for less than 4 years should be informed that the risk of osteonecrosis is very small but cannot be completely eliminated **(Table 14.6).** Dental treatment can be conducted with normal protocol without delay or alteration.

  In general, these patients should be informed of the importance of good oral hygiene and regular dental care.

- **Patients at modest risk**

  Patients above the age of 65 who have been on anti-resorptives for more than 4 years should be considered to be at modest risk of development of osteonecrosis of the jaw **(Table 14.6).**

  Routine care should include emphasis on good oral hygiene and regular dental care.

  If oral infection is detected, aggressive treatment should be promptly instituted. Although there is no concrete data supporting the use of chlorhexidine mouthwash, it can be recommended.

  Non-surgical options should be considered and endodontic techniques with preservation of the dental root is generally preferred over total tooth extraction.

  If dental surgery is necessary, the patient should be informed of the small risk of development of osteonecrosis of the jaw.

  If a significant surgical intervention is necessary, the patient's physician should be consulted to see if a "drug holiday" of 2 months prior to the intervention is feasible. There is no concrete date to support or refute this recommendation.

  During intervention, one sextant should be addressed at a time, with the allowance of a 2-month interval before the next intervention.

TABLE 14.6 Minimizing risks of osteonecrosis of the jaw in patients on anti-resorptives

Low risk (<4 years of therapy with no clinical risks)
Inform patient that the risk of osteonecrosis is very small but cannot be completely eliminated
No alteration or delay in planned dental intervention
Good oral hygiene
Regular dental care
Modest risk (>4 years of therapy with or without clinical risks)
Inform patient of small risk of osteonecrosis
Good oral hygiene
Regular dental care
Aggressive treatment of infection
0.12% chlorhexidine mouthwash
Consider non-surgical options - Endodontic techniques with preservation of the dental root preferred over total tooth extraction
Discuss risks prior to implant placement or surgery
Treat one sextant or tooth at a time, where feasible, and allow for a 2-month interval before next intervention
Should consider "drug holiday" for 2 months prior to intervention, if feasible, and restarted when osseous healing has occurred. (No data to support or refute)

- **Patients at high risk**

  Patients receiving high dose intravenous anti-resorptives or anti-angiogenic agents are at extremely high risk for development of osteonecrosis of the jaw, particularly with procedures that would cause significant bone trauma.

  These patients should be informed of the high risk of development of osteonecrosis with dental interventions. They should be recommended to follow aggressive protocols for good oral hygiene and regular dental care. Infection should be aggressively addressed **(Table 14.7).**

  Prior to any dental surgery, the patient's physician should be informed of the concerns over osteonecrosis of the jaw and, if feasible, a "drug holiday" of 2 months would be desirable. It is understood that a treatment plan may not permit the "drug holiday".

  Endodontic procedure is preferred over extraction, when feasible. Dental procedures should be carried out as atraumatically as possible. Teeth extraction should be undertaken only when the tooth mobility is 3 or greater. Dental implants should be avoided in these instances.

  In general, chlorhexidine mouthwash can be prescribed to be used 3-4 times a day.

TABLE 14.7 Management of patients at on anti-resorptives or anti-angiogenic agents for treatment of cancer

High risk	
Inform patient of risks	Recommended
Good oral hygiene	Recommended
Regular dental care	Recommended
Aggressive treatment of infection	Recommended
Endodontic procedure preferred over extraction	+
Extract teeth only when the mobility is 3 or greater	+
Atraumatic tooth extraction	+
0.12% chlorhexidine mouthwash	+
Drug holiday (stopping drug)	No data

5. Management of osteonecrosis of the jaw

Management of osteonecrosis of the jaw is largely supportive **(Table 14.8).** It is important to stop the offending anti-resorptive or anti-angiogenic agents if at all feasible.
Chlorhexidine rinses should be used 3–4 times a day.
Symptomatic sequestra should be removed surgically. Sharp edges of bone should be eliminated, and the wounds should be attempted with tension free closure.
Hyperbaric oxygen or ozone treatment have been used in severe cases.

TABLE 14.8 Management of osteonecrosis of the jaw

Treatment guidelines: general
0.12% chlorhexidine rinses 3–4 times a day
Aggressive treatment of infection
Surgical approach ◆ Removal of symptomatic sequestra ◆ Eliminate sharp edges of bone ◆ Tension free closure of wound Unfortunately, significant post-operative complications may result in more bone exposure
Hyperbaric oxygen +/– evidence
Ozone therapy +/– evidence

15 DENTAL EVALUATION AND MANAGEMENT OF THE PATIENT WITH HYPERTENSION

INTRODUCTION

Hypertension is the abnormal elevation of blood pressure above 120 mm Hg and/or the elevation of diastolic blood pressure above 80 mm of Hg. Approximately 66% of the dentist's adult population is affected by this disease under these stringent parameters. Hypertension adversely affects the patient by accelerating atherosclerosis. Untreated or inadequately treated hypertension is associated with increased morbidity and mortality from cerebrovascular disease, cardiovascular disease and peripheral vascular disease. Prospective studies have demonstrated that the control of hypertension is effective in the prevention of cerebrovascular disease, congestive heart failure and, to a lesser extent, coronary artery disease.

1. Medical evaluation of hypertension

It is clear that even mild hypertension is associated with progressive end-organ compromises. The guidelines have therefore reflected the need to control even mild hypertension through lifestyle modification. It is also clear that isolated systolic hypertension needs to be treated aggressively.

- **Morbidity of hypertension**

  Epidemiologic studies have indicated that for every 20 mm Hg increase in systolic blood pressure or 10 mm Hg increase in diastolic blood pressure, cardiovascular risk doubles. This has led to more aggressive guidelines for the management of hypertension.

- **Classification of hypertension**

  The epidemiologic data has led to continuing modification of the classification of hypertension.

The latest classification from the American Heart Association and American College of Cardiology **(Table 15.1)** has defined normal blood pressure as less than 120 mm Hg for systolic blood pressure and less than 80 mm Hg for diastolic blood pressure.
Blood pressure of 120–129 mm Hg of systolic blood pressure and less than 80 mm Hg of diastolic blood pressure is considered to be elevated blood pressure.
Blood pressure of 130–139 mm Hg of systolic blood pressure or 80–89 mm Hg of diastolic blood pressure is Stage 1 hypertension.
Blood pressure greater than 140 mm Hg of systolic blood pressure or greater than 90 mm Hg of diastolic blood pressure is Stage 2 hypertension.

TABLE 15.1 Classification of hypertension

Blood pressure (mm Hg)		
Systolic	**Diastolic**	
<120	and <80	Normal
120–129	and <80	Elevated blood pressure
130–139	or 80–89	Stage 1 hypertension
>140	or >90	Stage 2 hypertension

The classification is designed to heighten awareness of the importance of even minor degrees of elevation of blood pressure.

- **Importance of isolated systolic hypertension: a change in paradigm**
  The current guidelines also heighten the importance of isolated systolic hypertension (for instance, blood pressure of 170/70 mm Hg). Previously, more emphasis was placed on diastolic elevations, current data indicate that systolic hypertension is a significant factor for end organ damage. Isolated systolic hypertension is particularly common in patients above the age of 60. On the basis of the current evidence, the guidelines recommend a major paradigm shift in urging that isolated systolic hypertension becomes the major criterion for the diagnosis, staging and therapeutic management of hypertension, particularly in middle-aged and older patients.

2. Medical management of patients with hypertension

For patients with a mild elevation of blood pressure (120–129 mm Hg systolic and less than 80 mm Hg diastolic), the patients should be managed with lifestyle modifications: salt restriction, potassium supplementation, exercise, Dietary Approaches to Stop Hypertension (DASH) diet weight reduction and limited alcohol intake are recommended **(Table 15.2).**

For patients with Stage 1 or Stage 2 hypertension, the goal is to treat to 125–135 mm Hg systolic blood pressure and 80 mm Hg diastolic blood pressure.
In addition to lifestyle modification, medications such as diuretics, angiotensin-converting enzyme inhibitors (ACEIs), angiotensin receptor blockers (ARBs) or calcium channel blockers (CCBs) can be prescribed **(Table 15.2).**
Medical regimen is escalated monthly until the patient is at goal.
As long as the patient is asymptomatic, blood pressure lower than goal is acceptable.

TABLE 15.2 Treatment strategies for hypertension

Lifestyle changes: salt restriction, potassium supplement, unless contraindicated exercise, weight reduction, DASH diet and limited alcohol intake
Treat with diuretics, ACEIs (ACE Inhibitors), ARBs (Angiotensin Receptor Blockers) or calcium channel blocker (CCBs)
Continue to escalate medical regimen monthly until patient is at goal
As long as the patient is asymptomatic, blood pressure lower than goal is reasonable

3. Dental evaluation and management of the patient with hypertension

Dentists should play a major role in the detection of hypertension because they routinely see patients for multiple visits and semi-annual checkups. Monitoring a patient's blood pressure is an easy task and an important aspect of comprehensive dental-medical care because patients with hypertension are often asymptomatic.
In addition to playing a critical role in the screening process for hypertension, the dentist should also know how hypertension can complicate dental therapy. Poorly controlled blood pressure can acutely precipitate angina, congestive heart failure or, rarely, a cerebrovascular event such as a stroke or cerebral hemorrhage.

- **Patients with mild elevation of blood pressure and Stage 1 hypertension**
  Patients with mild elevation of blood pressure (120–129 mm Hg systolic and <80 mm Hg diastolic) and Stage 1 hypertension (130–139 mm Hg systolic or 80–89 mm Hg diastolic) can tolerate all nonsurgical and simple surgical procedures using normal protocol. It is important to establish good patient rapport and the appointments should be kept short. Multiple extractions or quadrant or full arch periodontal and oral surgery may require use of various sedation techniques **(Table 15.3).**

TABLE 15. 3 Dental management of patients with mild elevation of blood pressure and Stage 1 hypertension

Stress reduction	Patient rapport Short appointments
Sedation protocol	Consider oral conscious sedation Consider use of nitrous oxide

- **Patients with Stage 2 hypertension**

  Patients with Stage 2 hypertension should have their regimen reviewed by their physicians to see if control can be optimized,

  Patients wither Stage 2 hypertension will benefit from good patient rapport and short appointments. Nonsurgical procedures can be performed using normal protocols. Advanced crown and bridge and all simple surgical procedures should be carried out using adjunctive sedation techniques. Vasoconstrictors should be limited to less than 2 carpules of local anesthetics containing 1:100,000 epinephrine or 1:20,000 levonordefrin **(Table 15.4)**.

TABLE 15.4 Management of patients with Stage 2 hypertension

Stress reduction	Patient rapport Short appointments
Sedation protocol	Consider oral conscious sedation Consider use of nitrous oxide
Limit use of vasoconstrictors	Less than 2 carpules of local anesthetics containing 1:100,000 epinephrine or 1:20,000 levonordefrin
All non-surgical and simple surgical procedures	Normal protocol
Complex prosthetic and surgical procedures	Strongly consider sedation protocols

- **Patients with severe, uncontrolled hypertension (systolic blood pressure in excess of 160 mm Hg or diastolic blood pressure greater than 100 mm Hg)**

  The patient should only receive an examination and be referred to a physician for further medical management prior to additional dental care. Under a monitored environment, palliative care can be undertaken. However, vasoconstrictors are absolutely contraindicated, which clearly limits the scope of the dental intervention.

  Complex prosthetics and surgical procedures should not be undertaken **(Table 15.5)**.

TABLE 15.5 Management of patients with severe uncontrolled hypertension

Management
Dental examination only
Palliative care under monitored environment
Stress reduction is of paramount importance
Complex prosthetics and surgical procedures should not be undertaken
Vasoconstrictors absolutely contraindicated

4. Patients taking calcium channel blockers

Calcium channel blockers are a relatively frequent cause of gingival hyperplasia. Clinically, patients commonly present with enlargement of the marginal and papillary gingivae, which mimics the presentation of hyperplasia induced by phenytoin. Because hyperplastic changes in the gingiva often predispose to plaque accumulation and limit oral hygiene, a superimposed inflammatory process is often present.

Gingival hyperplasia appears to be most pronounced with nifedipine, less with the most commonly prescribed calcium channel blocker amlodipine and least with isradipine, which is rarely prescribed.

The major dental consideration for patients taking calcium channel blocker is maintenance of periodontal health. Because inflammation is likely to exacerbate gingival changes, aggressive oral hygiene and frequent professional maintenance are critical.

When possible, margins of fixed restorations should be placed supragingivally. Gingival resection may be required to eliminate overgrown tissue.

In severe, recurrent cases, or in patients who have difficulty with home care, in consultation with the patient's physicians, alternate medications may be necessary.

5. Use of vasoconstrictors in the hypertensive patient

One of the most discussed issues is the use of local anesthetics with vasoconstrictors. Even judicious use of vasoconstrictors can result in elevation of serum epinephrine with resultant elevation of blood pressure and/or arrhythmia.

It is clear that limitation to 2 carpules of 1:100,000 or epinephrine or 1:20,000 of levonordefrin or 4 carpules of 1: 200,000 of epinephrine is generally safe for the hypertensive patient **(Table 15.6).** This can result in a change in the treatment plan and breaking up long procedures into several phases.

TABLE 15.6 Maximal one-time dose of vasoconstrictor in patients with cardiac contraindications

Vasoconstrictor	Maximal dose
Epinephrine 1:50,000	AVOID
Epinephrine 1:100,000	2 carpules
Epinephrine 1:200,000	4 carpules
Levonordefrin 1:20,000	2 carpules

16 DENTAL EVALUATION AND MANAGEMENT OF THE PATIENT WITH ISCHEMIC HEART DISEASE

INTRODUCTION

Ischemic heart disease is the result of myocardial oxygen demand exceeding that of available oxygen supply as a result of coronary artery atherosclerosis.
Ischemic heart disease can be symptomatic with chest pain (angina), dyspnea on exertion (congestive heart failure) or, rarely, arrhythmia.
Ischemic heart disease can be managed medically. However, increasingly, percutaneous intervention of the coronary arteries may be deployed.
Medications used to manage ischemic heart disease can have dental implications. Patients with percutaneous cardiac interventions are often on anti-platelet agents, which carries significant implications for dental interventions.

1. Medical evaluation of ischemic heart disease

In a patient presenting with chest pain or dyspnea on exertion, a medical history, a physical examination and an electrocardiogram are generally performed.
If ischemic heart disease is clinically suspected, exercise stress tests or a stress echocardiogram can better define the nature and magnitude of the disease. In some patients, a cardiac CT angiogram may help define the coronary anatomy. In instances of high suspicion and in suitable patients, coronary catheterization and intervention might be done.

- **Stable angina**

  Angina, chest pain as a result of ischemic heart disease, may be the first indication of inadequate blood supply. The pain is classically described as a squeezing pressure in the substernal area, with radiation to the left side of the jaw and down the medial aspect of the left arm.

Stable angina is characterized by infrequent episodes that are precipitated by stress or exertion and are relieved by rest. These episodes last minutes and resolve spontaneously or are promptly relieved by nitroglycerin.

- **Unstable angina**
  Unstable angina is characterized by increasing frequency of episodes and severity of chest pain. The pain is often longer in duration and precipitated by minimal exertion or stress. At times, patients may have angina even at rest. Unstable angina is often a result of plaque rupture that can rapidly progress to a myocardial infarction. Unstable angina is a medical emergency and patients should immediately be referred for medical evaluation and management.

- **Dyspnea on exertion**
  In some patient, the inadequacy of oxygen supply to the heart can result in cardiac dysfunction, pulmonary congestion and dyspnea with exertion. This resolves with rest or with nitroglycerin.
  Since there are multiple reasons for dyspnea on exertion, one has to have a high index of suspicion to be able to diagnose ischemic heart disease with this presentation.

- **Atypical chest pain**
  Some patients can present with chest pain that is not typical. Pain may be located in the epigastrium or even the right side of the chest. Pain may have atypical radiation. One has to have a high index of suspicion and a low threshold to investigate possible ischemic heart disease in these instances.

2. Medical management of patients with ischemic heart disease

As indicated previously, unstable angina is a medical emergency and would prompt urgent cardiac catheterization and intervention.

- **Medical management of ischemic heart disease**
  Beta blockers and long-acting nitrates are the mainstay of medical management of ischemic heart disease.
  In patients with dyspnea on exertion, a diuretic may be added to optimize fluid management.
  All patients with ischemic heart disease should carry nitroglycerin. If symptoms occur, they are instructed to place the medication sublingually. Patients may need a second nitroglycerin if symptoms are not relieved after 5 minutes. If symptoms persist after a second nitroglycerin, the patient should immediately be referred to the emergency room.

- **Percutaneous coronary intervention**

  Increasingly, percutaneous coronary interventions are performed in patients with symptomatic ischemic heart disease. This would involve the use of a percutaneously guided balloon placed at the point of coronary artery stenosis. The balloon is inflated at 2 atmospheric pressure to flatten the atheromatous plaques. In rare instances, the balloon angioplasty might be the only procedure done, if the patient is deemed to be at high risk for anti-platelet therapy.

  In the vast majority of the instances, however, a stent would be placed after the balloon angioplasty to keep the area patent. Depending upon the device deployed, varying periods of dual anti-platelet therapy would be necessary.

  In instances where the coronary artery is completely occluded, atherectomy may be employed. This would involve a rotating blade creating a channel through the occluded vessel. A basket is placed downstream to collect the debris from the cutting blade. A stent is then placed in the open channel. The patient will require dual anti-platelet therapy.

  The specific stent deployed is generally dictated by the clinical situation:

  - **Bare metal stents** are used in instances where there are concerns over extended use of dual anti-platelet therapy. The hope is that the stent would be endothelialized over time. Although dual anti-platelet therapy is still necessary initially, this can be converted to single anti-platelet therapy after 6 months. However, progressive endothelialization of the stents can result in restenosis, making them less attractive than drug-eluting stents.
  - **Drug-eluting stents** have a drug embedded in the material coating the stent that prevents endothelialization. These are the most commonly stents used because the likelihood of restenosis is significantly decreased with drug-eluting stents. However, if anti-platelet drugs are withdrawn prematurely in these patients, the stent can thrombose. It is therefore recommended that double anti-platelet therapy be maintained for 12 months after stent placement.
  - **Bioresorbable vascular scaffolds,** where the substance in these devices would be resorbed over time, have made an initial appearance, but their use is currently on hold clinically because of efficacy concerns. It is anticipated that other iterations of these scaffolds will be in clinical use.

3. Surgical management of ischemic heart disease

Some patients may not be candidates for percutaneous interventions and may proceed to surgical intervention.

Patients after coronary artery bypass graft (CABG) are generally still on medical management and would need assessment of recurrent symptoms of ischemic heart disease. Limitation of vasoconstrictors should be dictated by the functional status of the patient at the time of the planned dental intervention.

4. Dental evaluation and management of the patient with ischemic heart disease

Dentists should be familiar with the medications the patients are on and the percutaneous procedures the patients have had.
The stability of the cardiac status should be assessed every session. If there are changes in symptoms, the patient should be referred to their physician for evaluation prior to any dental intervention.
Patients on dual anti-platelet therapy need to be identified and dental therapy appropriately adjusted. There will be excessive bleeding on dual anti-platelet therapy. In the appropriate patient, it would be prudent to inquire about the possibility of converting dual anti-platelet inhibition to single anti-platelet therapy. This does mean that the dentist should be familiar with the different stents the patient might have since the duration of dual anti-platelet therapy differs for the different stents.
One issue that invariably arises while considering dental procedures in patients with ischemic heart disease is the restriction of use of vasoconstrictors in local anesthetics.

- **Use of vasoconstrictors in patients with ischemic heart disease**

  One of the most discussed issues is the use of local anesthetics with vasoconstrictors in patients with ischemic heart disease. Even judicious use of vasoconstrictors can result in elevation of serum epinephrine with resultant elevation of blood pressure and/or arrhythmia.
  It is clear that limitation to 2 carpules of 1:100,000 or epinephrine or 1:20,000 of levonordefrin or 4 carpules of 1: 200,000 of epinephrine is generally safe for the cardiac patient **(Table 16.1).** This can result in a change in treatment plan and breaking up long procedures into several phases.

TABLE 16.1 Maximal one-time dose of vasoconstrictor in patients with cardiac contraindications

Epinephrine 1:50,000	AVOID
Epinephrine 1:100,000	2 carpules
Epinephrine 1:200,000	4 carpules
Levonordefrin 1:20,000	2 carpules

- **Dental management of patients with stable angina on medical management**

  In a patient with a history of ischemic heart disease, the stability of the symptoms should be assessed at each session.
  Patients with stable angina should have short appointments to minimize stress. All non-surgical and simple surgical procedures can be done with normal protocol **(Table 16.2).** Sedation protocol should be considered for complex prosthetic and oral surgical procedures (Chapter 45).

If the patient has functional capacity of greater than 4 METS, local anesthetics should be used judiciously.
If the patient has functional status of less than 4 METS, the dentist should limit the use of vasoconstrictor to 2 carpules.

TABLE 16.2 Dental management of patients with stable angina on medical management

Stress reduction	Patient rapport; short appointments
Limit use of vasoconstrictors	Limit use of vasoconstrictor to 2 carpules of 1:100,000 of epinephrine or 1:20,000 of levonordefrin
All non-surgical and simple surgical procedures	Normal protocol
Complex prosthetic and oral surgical procedures	Consider sedation protocol
Sedation protocol	Consider oral conscious sedation Consider use of nitrous oxide

- **Dental management of patients with bare metal stents**

In a patient with a history of a bare metal stent, the patient should be assessed at each session that the cardiac status is stable **(Table 16.3).**
Asymptomatic patients should have short appointments to minimize stress.
All non-surgical and simple surgical procedures can be done with normal protocol.
Complex prosthetic and oral surgical procedures should be avoided during the initial 6 months after the stent placement. Sedation protocol should be considered for these procedures after the first 6 months (Chapter 45).
If the patient has functional capacity of greater than 4 METS, local anesthetics should be used judiciously.
If the patient has functional status of less than 4 METS, the dentist should limit the use of vasoconstrictor to 2 carpules.
Patients with bare metal stents are generally on dual anti-platelet therapy for the first 6 months. Some may still be on dual therapy beyond the initial 6 months when the dentist may be considering complex surgical procedures. The dentist should consult the patient's cardiologist to see if aspirin can be stopped for 7 days prior to the planned dental procedure. Dual anti-platelet therapy can be resumed after the dental procedures.

TABLE 16.3 Management of patients with bare metal stents

Stress reduction	Patient rapport; short appointments Consider sedation protocol
Limit use of vasoconstrictors	Limit use of vasoconstrictor to 2 carpules of 1:100,000 of epinephrine or 1:20,000 of levonordefrin
All non-surgical and simple surgical procedures	Normal protocol
Complex prosthetic and oral surgical procedures	Avoid during the first 6 months Consider sedation protocol
Antibiotic premedication	Not indicated
Anti-platelet therapy	Patient should be off of anti-platelet agent except for ASA therapy beyond the first 6 months *Otherwise, consult physician about feasibility of holding ASA if the patient is on dual therapy*

- **Management of patients with drug-eluting stents**

  Management of the patient with drug-eluting stents is similar to management of the patient with bare-metal stents, except the duration of dual anti-platelet therapy is 12 months as opposed to 6 months.

  In a patient with a history of a drug-eluting stent, the patient should be assessed at each session that the cardiac status is stable.

  Asymptomatic patients should have short appointments to minimize stress.

  All non-surgical and simple surgical procedures can be done with normal protocol.

  Complex prosthetic and oral surgical procedures should be avoided during the initial 12 months after the stent placement. Sedation protocol should be considered for these procedures after the first 12 months (Chapter 45).

  If the patient has functional capacity of greater than 4 METS, local anesthetics should be used judiciously.

  If the patient has functional status of less than 4 METS, the dentist should limit the use of vasoconstrictor to 2 carpules.

Patients with drug-eluting stents are generally on dual anti-platelet therapy for the first 12 months.
Some may still be on dual therapy beyond the initial 12 months when the dentist may be considering dental surgery. The dentist should consult the patient's cardiologist to see if aspirin can be stopped for 7 days prior to planned dental procedure. Dual anti-platelet therapy can be resumed after the dental procedures.

- **Management of patients after coronary artery bypass graft**

A patient who has had a coronary artery bypass graft should be assessed at each session that the cardiac status is stable.
No elective dental surgery should be undertaken during the first 6 months after coronary artery bypass surgery to allow for stabilization of the cardiac status.
Six months after the cardiac surgery, asymptomatic patients should have short appointments to minimize stress.
All non-surgical and simple surgical procedures can be done with normal protocol.
Sedation protocol should be considered for complex prosthetic and oral surgical procedures (Chapter 45).
If the patient has functional capacity of greater than 4 METS, local anesthetics should be used judiciously.
If the patient has functional status of less than 4 METS, the dentist should limit the use of vasoconstrictor to 2 carpules.

5. Patients taking calcium channel blockers

Some patients with ischemic heart disease may be on calcium channel blockers.
Calcium channel blockers are a relatively frequent cause of gingival hyperplasia. Clinically, patients commonly present with enlargement of the marginal and papillary gingivae, which mimics the presentation of hyperplasia induced by phenytoin. Because hyperplastic changes in the gingiva often predispose to plaque accumulation and limit oral hygiene, a superimposed inflammatory process is often present.
Gingival hyperplasia appears to be most pronounced with nifedipine, less with the most commonly prescribed calcium channel blocker amlodipine and least with isradipine, which is rarely prescribed.
The major dental consideration for patients taking calcium channel blocker is maintenance of periodontal health. Because inflammation is likely to exacerbate gingival changes, aggressive oral hygiene and frequent professional maintenance are critical.
When possible, margins of fixed restorations should be placed supragingivally. Gingival resection may be required to eliminate overgrown tissue.
In severe, recurrent cases or in patients who have difficulty with home care, in consultation with the patient's physicians, alternate medications may be necessary.

17 DENTAL EVALUATION AND MANAGEMENT OF THE PATIENT WITH A HISTORY OF MYOCARDIAL INFARCTION

INTRODUCTION

Myocardial infarction occurs when cardiac ischemia results in damage of the myocardium. Patients with a history of myocardial infarction are more prone to recurrent ischemia and infarction, arrhythmia and congestive heart failure.
Previous American Heart Association (AHA) guidelines recommended that any dental surgery within 6 months of myocardial infarction should be avoided due to the high risk of complications during this period. The emerging evidence now advocates that **no elective dental care should be given within 30 days of the myocardial infarction.**

1. Dental evaluation of the patient with a history of myocardial infarction

Specific information should be ascertained from the medical history and in consultation with the patient's physician:

Medical history

- Date of myocardial infarction
- Extent of myocardial infarction
- Intervention: placement of stents during the myocardial infarction
- Complications including:
    - Residual ischemia
    - Decreased ejection fraction
    - Arrhythmia
    - Congestive heart failure

Medications the patient is on

- A full list of medications will give you a better sense of the magnitude of the myocardial infarction and the complications thereof.

2. Dental management of the patient with a history of myocardial infarction

All elective dental interventions should be avoided during the first 30 days after myocardial infarction.

General principles of dental management of patient after myocardial infarction (Table 17.1):

- The stability of the cardiac status should be assessed every session.
- If there are changes in symptoms, the patient should be referred to their physician for evaluation prior to any dental intervention.
- Avoid elective dental procedures within the first 30 days after myocardial infarction.
- Patients should have short appointments to minimize stress.
- All non-surgical and simple surgical procedures can be done with normal protocol (Table 17.1).
- Sedation protocol should be considered for complex prosthetic and oral surgical procedures (Chapter 45).

TABLE 17.1 Dental management of the patient with a history of myocardial infarction

Stress reduction	Patient rapport; short appointments
Limit use of vasoconstrictors	Limit use of vasoconstrictor to 2 carpules of 1:100,000 of epinephrine or 1:20,000 of levonordefrin
All non-surgical and simple surgical procedures	Normal protocol
Complex prosthetic and oral surgical procedures	Consider sedation protocol
Sedation protocol	Consider oral conscious sedation Consider use of nitrous oxide

3. Use of vasoconstrictors in the patient with a history of myocardial infarction

One of the most discussed issues is the use of local anesthetics with vasoconstrictors in patients with cardiac issues (Table 17.2).

- Even judicious use of vasoconstrictors can result in the elevation of serum epinephrine with resultant elevation of blood pressure and/or arrhythmia.
- It is clear that limitation to 2 carpules of 1:100,000 or epinephrine or 1:20,000 of levonordefrin or 4 carpules of 1: 200,000 of epinephrine is generally safe for the cardiac patient.
- This can result in change in the treatment plan and breaking up long procedures into several phases.

TABLE 17.2 Maximal one-time dose of vasoconstrictor in the patient after myocardial infarction

Epinephrine 1:50,000	AVOID
Epinephrine 1:100,000	2 carpules
Epinephrine 1:200,000	4 carpules
Levonordefrin 1:20,000	2 carpules

4. Medications with dental implications in the patient with a history of myocardial infarction

Many medications the patient may be taking after a myocardial infarction have dental implications. The dental professional should work closely with the patient's physician to try to optimize the care of the patient.

Single anti-platelet therapy after myocardial infarction

- Unless there is a medical contraindication, the patient is on single anti-platelet inhibition with aspirin indefinitely after myocardial infarction.
- Dental procedures can be carried out with careful attention to hemostasis.

Dual anti-platelet therapy after myocardial infarction

- If the patient had a stent placed during the myocardial infarction, dual anti-platelet therapy may be prescribed.
- Generally, patients can be converted to single anti-platelet therapy after 6 months.
- Patients with drug-eluting stents may be on dual anti-platelet therapy for a much longer period of time.
- In instances where there may be concerns over excessive bleeding, the dentist should confer with the cardiologist as to the feasibility of converting dual therapy to single therapy transiently.
- If it is deemed feasible, aspirin should be held for 7 days prior to the planned procedure. Clopidogrel or ticagrelor should be continued.
- Dual anti-platelet therapy should be resumed immediately following the procedure.

Calcium Channel Blockers

- Some patients may be placed on calcium channel blockers after myocardial infarction.
- Calcium channel blockers are a relatively frequent cause of gingival hyperplasia. Clinically, patients commonly present with enlargement of the marginal and papillary gingivae, which mimics the presentation of hyperplasia induced by phenytoin. Because hyperplastic changes in the gingiva often predispose to plaque accumulation and limit oral hygiene, a superimposed inflammatory process is often present.

- Gingival hyperplasia appears to be most pronounced with nifedipine, less with the most commonly prescribed calcium channel blocker amlodipine and least with isradipine, which is rarely prescribed.
- The major dental consideration for patients taking calcium channel blocker is maintenance of periodontal health.
- Because inflammation is likely to exacerbate gingival changes, aggressive oral hygiene and frequent professional maintenance are critical.
- When possible, margins of fixed restorations should be placed supra-gingivally. Gingival resection may be required to eliminate overgrown tissue.
- In severe, recurrent cases, or in patients who have difficulty with home care, in consultation with the patient's physicians, alternate medications may be necessary.

Guidelines for dental evaluation and management of the patient with a history of myocardial infarction have changed to avoiding procedures for the 30 days after the myocardial infarction from the previous AHA guidelines of 6 months. This will greatly facilitate planning of dental interventions. However, care should be exercised to avoid complications, and close collaboration with the medical professionals is of critical importance.

18 DENTAL EVALUATION AND MANAGEMENT OF THE PATIENT WITH HEART FAILURE

INTRODUCTION

Heart failure is the consequence of inadequate cardiac output to deliver amounts of oxygenated blood to meet the metabolic demand of the body.
Most frequently, patients with heart failure will have dyspnea on exertion, progressing to increasing functional compromises as a result of decreased cardiac output.
Cardiac function is usually measured by the ejection fraction of the left ventricle, which measures the percentage of blood leaving the chamber with every cardiac contraction. Ejection fraction can be accurately assessed by an echocardiogram. Normal ejection fraction is in the 45% to 65% range.
Compromised ejection fraction will create compromise in cardiac output. However, a patient with a stiff ventricle can have inadequate cardiac output although the ejection fraction is not compromised.

- **Heart failure with decreased ejection fraction**
  Heart failure may be due to myocardial compromise as a result of ischemic heart disease with a decrease in the ejection fraction (ischemic cardiomyopathy).
  Valvular disease such as mitral regurgitation or aortic stenosis can result in compromised cardiac performance.
  Rarely, decreased ejection fraction may be the result of viral myocarditis or an infiltrative disease affecting the heart such as amyloidosis (dilated cardiomyopathy).

- **Heart failure with preserved ejection fraction**
  With aggressive intervention for ischemic heart disease, increasing numbers of people with heart failure have preserved ejection fraction (heart failure with preserved ejection

fraction). These patients have a stiffened myocardium as a result of long-standing hypertension with resultant diastolic dysfunction. Rarely, the compromise may be a result of infiltrative disease of the myocardium such as amyloidosis.

The dentist should be aware of the increasing prevalence of heart failure, the different modalities of intervention and their effects on dental therapeutics.

1. Medical evaluation of heart failure

In a patient presenting with dyspnea on exertion, peripheral edema and progressive functional compromise. a medical history, a physical examination and an electrocardiogram are generally performed.

If there is clinical suspicion of heart failure, echocardiogram is the important next diagnostic test. This will provide information about the left ventricular ejection fraction and the function of the mitral and aortic valves.

Depending upon the clinical presentation, stress test (stress thallium or echo stress test) and cardiac CT angiogram may be performed. When clinically indicated, the patient may proceed to cardiac catheterization. During the cardiac angiogram, the pressures in the various chambers can be determined. An elevated wedge pressure is usually seen in patients with heart failure. Angioplasty and stent placement may be deployed to reverse coronary disease that may be the cause of the cardiac compromise.

In selected instances, myocardial biopsy might be done on the right ventricular wall to make the diagnosis of myocarditis or infiltrative cardiomyopathy such as amyloidosis.

- **Ejection fraction**

  On echocardiogram and on cardiac catheterization, the left ventricular ejection fraction can be accurately determined. **Table 18.1** delineates the significance of the ejection fraction obtained during these studies.

TABLE 18.1 Clinical significance of ejection fraction

>45%	Normal ejection fraction
40-45%	Mild compromise
30-40%	Moderate compromise
<30%	Severe compromise

- **Functional status of the patient**

  In addition to quantification of ejection fraction, the functional status of the patient should be characterized. One commonly used classification is the one put out by the New York Heart Association **(Table 18.2).**

TABLE 18.2 New York Heart Association (NYHA) classification of heart failure

Severity of heart failure		
Mild HF	NYHA Class II	Mild compromise of activity
	NYHA Class III	Moderate compromise of activity
Severe HF	NYHA Class IV	Severe compromise of activity; cannot walk up one flight of stairs

2. Medical management of patients with heart failure

Patients with acute decompensation are often managed as an inpatient. A variety of therapeutic options are available for patients with chronic congestive heart failure.

- **Lifestyle modification**

In general, patients with congestive heart failure are placed on a low salt diet. A healthy diet to promote optimization of weight is prescribed. Smoking cessation is of critical importance. Cardiac rehabilitation programs can tailor-make an exercise and weight reduction protocol.

- **Guideline-directed medical therapies (GDMT)**

In patients with heart failure, guidelines are well established by multiple professional societies including the American Heart Association/American College of Cardiology/Heart Failure Society of America, the European Society of Cardiology and the Canadian and the Japanese Societies of Cardiology.

Four classes of medications (Table 18.3) are used in guideline-directed medical therapies:

- **Medications acting on the renin-angiotensin system:**
  - **Angiotensin converting enzyme inhibitors (ACEIs)**
  - **Angiotensin-receptor blockers (ARBs) or**
  - **Angiotensin receptor/neprilysin inhibitor (ARNI)**

Interruption of the renin-angiotensin pathway is the foundation of management of congestive heart failure with reduced ejection fraction:

Any ACE inhibitors or ARBs can be titrated according to the patient's blood pressure. Additionally, agents can interfere with the neprilysin receptor, used in combination with an ARB/ARNI commonly used is sacubitril/valsartan (Entresto).

- **Beta blockers**

Cardioselective beta blockers are commonly used:
carvedilol, metoprolol or bisoprolol can be increased to maximal dose as tolerated.

- **Aldosterone antagonists**
  Spironolactone or eplironone is generally used.

- **Sodium-glucose cotransporter-2 (SGLT2) inhibitors**
  Medications such empagliflozin (Jardiance) or dapagliflozin (Farxiga) are used in GDMT. Chronic elimination of sodium is clearly of great benefit in management of congestive heart failure.
  In general, patients are on combinations of these medications, titrated to optimal doses. These guidelines have significantly improved the mortality and quality of life of patients with chronic congestive heart failure.
  Other medications such as diuretics and vasodilators are also important in management of selected patients.

TABLE 18.3 Common medications for guideline-directed medical therapy

Cardioselective beta blockers	Bisoprolol (Zebeta) Metoprolol (Toprol, Lopressor) Carvedilol (Coreg)
ACE inhibitors (ACEIs)	Lisinopril (Zestril, Prinivil) Enalopril (Vasotec) Ramipril (Altace) Quinapril (Accupril) Benazepril (Lotensin) Fosinopril (Monopril) Captopril (Captopril) Moexipril (Univasc) Perindopril (Aceon) Trandolapril (Mavik)
Angiotensin receptor blockers (ARBs)	Losartan (Cozaar) Irbesartan (Avapro) Valsartan (Diovan) Olmesartan (Benicar) Telmisartan (Micardis) Azilsartan (Edarbi) Candesartan (Atacand)
Combination drugs (ARNI)	Sacubitril/Valsartan (Ernesto)
Aldosterone antagonist	Spironolactone (Aldactone) Eplirenone (Inspra)
SGLT2 inhibitors	Dapafliglozin (Farxiga) Empagliflozin (Jardiance)

- **Cardiac resynchronization therapy (CRT) and implantable cardioverter defibrillator (ICD)**
  An implantable cardioverter defibrillator (ICD) is used for heart failure treatment when the patient is at high risk of sudden death from lethal arrhythmias. The risk is highest in those who already suffered from previous ventricular arrhythmic events but patients with low ejection fractions have also been shown to be at high risk. In general, ICD is considered in patients with ejection fraction of less than 35%. The defibrillator is implanted in the chest and continually monitors the heart's rhythm and would defibrillate rhythms such as ventricular tachycardia or ventricular fibrillation.

3. Dental evaluation and management of the patient with ischemic heart disease

Dentists should be familiar with the medications the patients are on and cardiac devices implanted. The underlying cardiac condition makes the patient a higher risk candidate for dental interventions and appropriate precautions should be taken.

- **Use of vasoconstrictors in patients with congestive heart failure**
  Vasoconstrictor should be limited to 2 carpules of 1:100,000 of epinephrine or 1:20,000 of levonordefrin or 4 carpules of 1:200,000 epinephrine for patients with ischemic heart disease.
  Since some of the dental procedures are lengthy, the local anesthetic can be spread out over time. Technical considerations such as mandibular blocks and use of different local anesthetics can help minimize total dose of vasoconstrictor used. It may even be necessary to change the dental plan to allow for shorter sessions in order to minimize local anesthetic use.

- **Dental management of patients with congestive heart failure**
  In a patient with a history of congestive heart failure, the stability of the symptoms should be assessed at each session.
  Patients with stable symptoms should have short appointments to minimize stress. All non-surgical and simple surgical procedures can be done with normal protocol **(Table 18.4).** Sedation protocol should be considered for complex prosthetic and oral surgical procedures (Chapter 45).
  In all instances, the dentist should limit the use of vasoconstrictor in a patient with congestive heart failure.

TABLE 18.4 Dental management of patients with congestive heart failure

Stress reduction	Patient rapport; short appointments
Limit use of vasoconstrictors	Limit use of vasoconstrictor to 2 carpules of 1:100,000 of epinephrine or 1:20,000 of levonordefrin
All non-surgical and simple surgical procedures	Normal protocol
Complex prosthetic and oral surgical procedures	Consider sedation protocol
Sedation protocol	Consider oral conscious sedation Consider use of nitrous oxide

- **Dental management of patients with CRT-ICD (Table 18.5)**

A number of studies have shown that some electronic dental devices may cause interference with implanted cardiac devices. There is conflicting evidence since most of the positive results come from in vitro studies. It is believed that human tissues should provide some shielding that cannot be accounted for in the in vitro studies. Nonetheless, caution should be exercised when electronic dental devises are used in these patients.

The newer cardiac devices are better shielded and are less susceptible to interference. In general, piezoelectric dental scalers are safer than magnetostrictive scalers. Electrosurgery devices have the highest potential of interference.

Electrosurgery units used to cauterize and remove tissue have been regarded by both the Heart Rhythm Society and the American Society of Anesthesiologists as the most common source of electromagnetic interference and stated that head and neck surgery region surgeries using monopolar equipment pose more of a risk for oversensing and damage to the CRT-ICD system. It is therefore reasonable to avoid use of monopolar electrosurgical units if possible.

From a practical standpoint, the closer the instruments are to the device, the more interference is expected. Proper use and distancing is therefore important in minimizing interference.

TABLE 18.5 Management of patients with CRT-ICD

Consider age of CRT-ICD	Devices placed within the past 5 years are better shielded and are less susceptible to interference
Limit use of vasoconstrictors	Patients with ICD should have limitation of vasoconstrictor use
All non-surgical and simple surgical procedures	Minor concerns with ultrasonic dental scalers: piezoelectric scalers are safer than magnetostriction devices Maximize distance to cardiac device
Complex prosthetic and oral surgical procedures	Minor concerns with apex locators and pulp testers Higher concerns with monopolar electrosurgical units used to remove and cauterize tissues; avoid use if possible
Antibiotic premedication	Not indicated
Positioning	Inasmuch as possible, maximize distance of instruments to the cardiac device

- **Medication-related concerns**

  Many of the medications used for management of congestive heart failure lower the blood pressure. It is therefore important to monitor the patient's vital signs during the dental procedures.

  Diuretics and SGLT2 inhibitors can cause volume depletion. One should be aware of the possibility of orthostatic hypotension and should get the patient up slowly after the dental procedure.

Congestive heart failure in increasing in incidence and prevalence. Understanding how to evaluate and manage this group of patients is of great importance in the optimal care of these patients.

19 MEDICAL EVALUATION AND MANAGEMENT OF THE PATIENT WITH DIABETES MELLITUS

In order to be able to render optimal dental care to patients with diabetes mellitus, it is important to understand the medical evaluation and management of patients with diabetes mellitus. Much of the testing and treatment of these patients will impact dental evaluation and management.

INTRODUCTION

Diabetes mellitus affects one out of eight patients presenting to the dental office. Patients with diabetes mellitus have increased risk of developing oral health complications. Equally importantly, poor oral health can complicate control of diabetes with significant systemic health implications.

- **Type 1 diabetes mellitus**

Type 1 diabetes mellitus is the result of the absolute inability of the pancreas to produce insulin. This is usually the result of an autoimmune disease that destroys the beta cells of the pancreas. About 10% of patients with diabetes are type 1.
Since they cannot produce insulin, treatment depends on various ways of delivering and monitoring efficacy of insulin therapy.
These patients tend to have more severe disease, more end-organ damage and more complicated management issues.

- **Type 2 diabetes mellitus**

Type 2 diabetes mellitus is the result of peripheral resistance to insulin produced. Patients tend to be overweight. Although the mainstay of management revolves around lifestyle modifications, many patients require additional treatment with a forever expanding number of options for blood sugar management.

The dentist should be aware of the increasing prevalence of diabetes mellitus, the different modalities of intervention and their effects on dental therapeutics.

1. Medical evaluation of patients with diabetes mellitus

Diabetes mellitus is generally detected during routine testing of a patient. In rare instances, patients may present with symptoms of polyuria, polydipsia and weight loss.

Diagnosis: HbA1c

In general, when diabetes is suspected because of symptoms or elevated blood sugar detected in a routine evaluation, we rely on hemoglobin A1c level to make the diagnosis of diabetes. Hemoglobin A1c provides us with an estimate of the average blood sugar level over the previous 60-90 days. It has replaced fasting blood sugars, post-prandial blood sugar and glucose tolerance test for diagnosis of diabetes mellitus.
Patients with normal blood sugar control generally have HbA1c levels close to 5.0%. Elevation of HbA1c denotes poor glycemic control. Poor control would result in increasing propensity for development of diabetic complications (Table 19.1).

TABLE 19.1 Hemoglobin A1c (HbA1c) and adequacy of control

Adequacy of control	
HbA1c ‹6.5% (BS 140 mg/dL)	Excellent control
HbA1c 6.5-8.5% (BS 140-200 mg/dL)	Marginal control
HbA1c ›8.5% (BS 200 mg/dL)	Poor control

Insulin level

In general, the clinical presentation is adequate to delineate type 1 from type 2 diabetes mellitus. On rare occasions, insulin levels might be helpful: patients with type 1 diabetes usually have a low endogenous level of insulin. This may fall further with the progression of disease.

2. Medical management of patients with type 1 diabetes mellitus

Because the patients with type 1 diabetes mellitus cannot produce adequate amount of insulin, management revolves around the various modes of delivery of insulin and monitoring of efficacy. The primary goal is to maintain blood sugars within a target range to prevent acute and long-term complications.

Lifestyle modification

In general, patients with type 1 diabetes mellitus are instructed on a diet and exercise regimen. Being able to adjust insulin regimen to the daily activities is important for the optimization of disease control.

Insulin therapy

Insulin therapy is the cornerstone of management of the patient with type 1 diabetes. Different forms of insulin (Table 19.2) have different onset of action and different duration of action. Different forms may be mixed and given at varying schedules to optimize blood sugar control. Insulin dosing is often governed by dietary intake and level of exercise.

TABLE 19.2 Insulin preparations, onset of action and duration of action

Insulin management		
Type	**Onset of action**	**Duration**
Ultra-rapid acting (Faster aspart)	0.1 to 0.2 hours	3-5 hours
Rapid acting (Lispro, Aspart, Glulisine)	0.15 to 0.35 hours	3-5 hours
Short acting (Regular)	0.5-1.0 hours	5-8 hours
Intermediate acting (NPH, NPL)	2-4 hours	4-12 hours
Long acting (Glargine, Detemir, Degludec)	2-4 hours	8-12 hours

Monitoring of blood sugar

Adequate control of blood sugar in the patient with type 1 diabetes mellitus is highly dependent upon accurate and frequent monitoring of blood sugar.

- **Finger stick:** traditional way of monitoring is the use of a lancet to obtain a droplet of blood from the tip of the finger and measuring the glucose level on a glucometer. Ideal control requires repeated finger sticks and patients with type 1 diabetes mellitus would often do four or more finger pricks per day to optimize adjustment of insulin dosing.
- **Continuous glucose monitoring:** an important development in the management of type 1 diabetes mellitus is the availability of devices inserted subcutaneously that can provide continuous (or near continuous) monitoring of blood sugars. The resulted blood sugars recorded in these devices can transmit the results to mobile devices such as a mobile phone via Bluetooth technology. These devices have revolutionized insulin management since the patient has up-to-the-minute blood sugars upon which they can make decisions about insulin dosing.

Administration of insulin

- **Multiple administration of insulin mixture:** in order to optimize blood sugar control, different forms of insulin are often mixed and administered multiple times a day.

- **Insulin pump:** continuous infusion pumps have been introduced to allow for continuous infusion of a low basal rate of insulin with the addition of boluses to cover expected increases in blood sugar associated with meals and with snacks. Advancement in this arena has resulted in very small pumps capable of continuous infusion of insulin over days. These pumps currently can be connected to mobile devices such as a mobile phone via Bluetooth technology to conveniently allow administration of correct insulin doses without having to carry additional monitors or infusion sets.

- **Closed loop system**
  With the miniaturization of both the continuous glucose monitoring devices and the insulin pump, it is now possible to have the glucose monitor directly regulate the amount of insulin to be infused. We now, in essence, can mimic pancreatic function with these external devices. It is therefore expected that patients with type 1 diabetes mellitus can now have very adequate control of their blood sugars, with the expectation that this will greatly improve the long-term prognosis of the type 1 diabetic.

- **Long-term disease monitoring**
  Type 1 diabetics are prone to small and large vessel disease and should be regularly monitored for development of diabetic retinopathy, nephropathy and peripheral neuropathy. They should be closely followed by their diabetologist, dietician, ophthalmologist and podiatrist regularly. If needed, they are referred to nephrology and neurology for specific sub-specialty needs.

3. Medical management of patients with type 2 diabetes mellitus

Because the patients with type 2 diabetes mellitus have peripheral insulin resistance, usually secondary to obesity, lifestyle modification is of paramount importance. In instances where lifestyle modification failed to control the blood sugar, oral hypoglycemic agents are prescribed. In some instances, patients with type 2 diabetes mellitus may have to have insulin therapy to achieve adequate control.

- **Lifestyle modification**
  In general, patients with type 2 diabetes mellitus are overweight and weight reduction can go a long way to optimizing control. It is critical that the patients are instructed on a diet and exercise program, both to optimize blood sugar control and to help with weight reduction. The program should be regularly reviewed and adjustments should be made to optimize a healthy diet.

- **Oral hypoglycemic drugs**
  There are innumerable drugs that can lower blood sugar **(Table 19.3).** The mainstay of oral hypoglycemic agent is metformin. Unless contraindicated, lifestyle modification and optimization of metformin use should be the pillars of management of patients with type 2 diabetes.

If lifestyle modification and metformin are unable to optimize blood sugar control, second line drugs can be added (Table 19.3).
Many of the second line therapies are costly, and some may involve weekly subcutaneous injections.

It should be stressed that some classes of agents have been shown to have additional end-organ protective (cardiac or renal) effects or a desirable side effect profile (weight loss). Many drugs are therefore used in arenas beyond just blood sugar control.

Therefore, the choice of second line agents is often dependent upon cost and desired secondary benefits. It is not unusual for a patient to be on multiple agents to optimize blood sugar control, and new drugs are arriving on the market rapidly that greatly increase the options.

TABLE 19.3 Oral hypoglycemics for management of type 2 diabetes mellitus (drugs in bold italics are gaining in use, often because of secondary effects)

Class	Drug
Biguanides *First line therapy*	***Metformin (Glucophage)***
Glucagon-like peptide-1 agonist *Reduces cardiovascular disease in patients with existing disease*	Exenatide (Byetta, Bydureon)
	Liraglutide (Victoza)
	Dulaglutide (Trulicity)
	Albiglutide (Tanzeum)
	Lixisenatide (Lyxumia)
SGLT2 inhibitors (sodium-glucose cotransporter-2 proteins) *Empagliflozin for cardiovascular benefits, particularly CHF* *Dapagliflozin for renal benefits*	Canagliflozin (Invokana)
	Dapagliflozin (Farxiga)
	Empagliflozin (Jardiance)
	Ertugliflozin (Steglatro, Segluromet, Steglujan)
	Ipragliflozin (Suglat)
Glucagon-like peptide-1 receptor agonist *Weight reduction*	***Semaglutide (Ozempic)***
Glucagon-like peptide-1 receptor agonist and glucose-dependent insulinotropic polypeptide receptor agonist *Weight reduction*	***Tirzepatide (Mounjaro)***
Second generation sulfonylureas *Less costly*	Glyburide (DiaBeta, Micronase)
	Glipizide (Glucotrol)
	Glimepiride (Amaryl)
	Gliclazide (Diamicron)

Cont'd

Cont'd

DPP-4 inhibitors (inhibitors of dipeptidyl peptidase 4) *Reduction of major adverse cardiovascular events*	Sitagliptin (Januvia)
	Saxagliptin (Onglyza)
	Linagliptin (Tradjenta)
	Vildagliptin (Galvus)
	Alogliptin (Nesina)
Alpha-glucosidase inhibitors	Acarbose (Precose)
	Miglitol (Glyset)
	Voglibose (Voglib)
	Pramlintide (Symlin)
Thiazolindediones (concern over cardiovascular safety)	Pioglitazone (Actos)
	Rosiglitazone (Avandia)
Meglitinide	Repaglinide (Prandin)
	Nateglinide (Starlix)
Insulin	

- **Insulin therapy**
  If lifestyle modification and oral hypoglycemic agents are not adequate for control of blood sugar, insulin therapy may be added.

- **Monitoring of blood sugar**
  Adequate control of blood sugar in the patient with type 2 diabetes mellitus is dependent upon accurate monitoring of blood sugar.
  - **Finger stick:** The traditional way of monitoring is the use of a lancet to obtain a droplet of blood from the tip of the finger and measuring the glucose level on a glucometer. Ideal control requires repeated finger sticks and patients with type 2 diabetes mellitus would often do four or more finger pricks per day to optimize adjustment of insulin dosing.
  - **Continuous glucose monitoring:** An important development in the management of type 2 diabetes mellitus is the availability of devices inserted subcutaneously that can provide continuous (or near continuous) monitoring of blood sugars. The resulted blood sugars recorded in these devices can transmit the results to mobile devices such as a mobile phone via Bluetooth technology. These devices have revolutionized diabetic management since the patient has up-to-the-minute blood sugars upon which they can make decisions about their diet and adequacy of control.
    Unfortunately, access to continuous glucose monitoring is not universal because of the cost incurred.

- **Long-term disease monitoring**

  Type 2 diabetics are prone to small vessel disease and should be regularly monitored for development of diabetic retinopathy, nephropathy and peripheral neuropathy. They should be closely followed by their diabetologist, dietician, ophthalmologist and podiatrist regularly.

  They are also susceptible to large vessel disease such as coronary artery disease, peripheral artery disease and cerebrovascular disease. If necessary, they are referred to nephrology, cardiology and neurology for specific sub-specialty needs.

  Understanding the medical evaluation and treatment of diabetes is critical for the dental evaluation and management of patients with either type 1 or type 2 diabetes mellitus.

4. Long-term complications of diabetes mellitus

Adequacy of control has enormous impact on development of long-term complications of diabetes.

From the dental standpoint, dental infections and periodontitis **(Table 19.4)** are more common in diabetic patients. These are accentuated with poor control. Poor oral health, in turn, would worsen diabetic control.

From the medical standpoint, large and small vessel disease can result in debilitating long-term complications:

Small vessel disease results in retinopathy, neuropathy and nephropathy: diabetes is the leading cause of blindness, non-traumatic amputation of limbs and end-stage renal disease.

Large vessel disease results in increased incidence of coronary artery disease, carotid artery disease, peripheral vascular disease and cerebrovascular disease.

TABLE 19.4 Complication of diabetes mellitus

Types of complications
Dental infection
Periodontitis
Retinopathy
Neuropathy
Nephropathy
Vasculopathy

20 DENTAL EVALUATION AND MANAGEMENT OF THE PATIENT WITH DIABETES MELLITUS

INTRODUCTION

Diabetes mellitus affects one out of eight patients presenting to the dental office. Patients with diabetes mellitus have increased risk of developing oral health complications. Equally importantly, poor oral health can complicate control of diabetes with significant systemic health implications.

- **Type 1 diabetes mellitus**
  Type 1 diabetes mellitus is the result of the absolute inability of the pancreas to produce insulin. This is usually the result of an autoimmune disease that destroys the beta cells of the pancreas. About 10% of patients with diabetes are type 1.
  Since they cannot produce insulin, treatment depends on various ways of delivering and monitoring efficacy of insulin therapy.
  These patients tend to have more severe disease, more end-organ damage and more complicated management issues.

- **Type 2 diabetes mellitus**
  Type 2 diabetes mellitus is the result of peripheral resistance to insulin produced. Patients tend to be overweight. Although the mainstay of management revolves around lifestyle modifications, many patients require additional treatment with a forever expanding number of options for blood sugar management.
  The dentist should be aware of the increasing prevalence of diabetes mellitus, the different modalities of intervention and their effects on dental therapeutics.

1. Dental evaluation of patients with diabetes mellitus

It is important to delineate the form of diabetes the patient has, the therapy being employed, the adequacy of diabetic control and the presence of vascular, renal, neurological or infectious complications.

Patients should be specifically asked about the duration of their disease, the frequency of occurrence of hypoglycemia, a history of ketoacidosis and diabetic-related hospitalizations.

- **Form of diabetes**

  This should be clearly delineated in the medical records since it has significant therapeutic implications.

- **Treatment modality**

  For patients on oral hypoglycemic agents, the specific medications they are on should be carefully recorded.

  For patients on insulin therapy, the type of insulin, the amount and timing of administration should be recorded.

  Special note should be made for patients on insulin pumps.

- **Assessing adequacy of control**

  The dentist should always ask the diabetic patient about their most recent hemoglobin A1c level. Hemoglobin A1c provides us with an estimate of the average blood sugar level over the previous 60-90 days. It has replaced fasting blood sugars, post-prandial blood sugar and glucose tolerance test for diagnosis of diabetes mellitus.

  Patients with normal blood sugar control generally have HbA1c levels close to 5.0%. Elevation of HbA1c denotes poor glycemic control. Poor control would result in increasing propensity for development of diabetic complications **(Table 20.1).**

  HbA1c should be used to help guide dental intervention. Poor control can result in substantive changes in therapeutic plans.

TABLE 20.1 Hemoglobin A1c (HbA1c) and adequacy of control

Adequacy of control	
HbA1c <6.5% (BS 140 mg/dL)	Excellent control
HbA1c 6.5-8.5% (BS 140-200 mg/dL)	Marginal control
HbA1c >8.5% (BS 200 mg/dL)	Poor control

2. Dental management of patients with diabetes mellitus: general guidelines

The primary goal should be to avoid untoward metabolic imbalances during dental therapy. Patients should be carefully instructed about their diet and their medications during the course of therapy so as to minimize problems related to either hypoglycemia or hyperglycemia. The dentist should also attempt to minimize stress and the risk of infection.

- **Scheduling of appointments**

  Inasmuch as possible, the patient should have as little interruption of their diet as possible in order to avoid hypoglycemia.

  The patient should be instructed to have a light, non-fatty breakfast and to have their normal medications at the normal appointed times.

  The patient should be scheduled as the first morning case of the day.

  The appointment should not exceed 3 hours so as not to interfere with oral intake at lunch.

- **Oral hypoglycemic agents**

  Patients should be instructed to take their normal dosage of oral hypoglycemic agents for all outpatient dental procedures.

- **Insulin therapy**

  Unless there is concern over alteration of meal timing, the patient should be instructed to have their normal dose of insulin.

  In instances where meal timing may be altered, the patient may be instructed to take half of the normal dose of insulin and to have a normal breakfast. The patient can be given the other half of the insulin dose when a normal diet is resumed after the dental procedures.

- **Insulin pump**

  Patients on an insulin pump should have a normal breakfast and a normal bolus of insulin with breakfast and be maintained on basal rate of infusion through the dental procedure.

- **Minimization of stress**

  The dentist should try to minimize stress to the diabetic patient in order to minimize glycemic perturbation. Whenever feasible, lengthy procedures should be spread over several shorter appointments. When appropriate, adjunctive sedation techniques such as oral conscious sedation, use of nitrous oxide and intravenous sedation should be considered.

- **Minimization of risk of infection**

  Diabetics are at increased risk of developing dental infections, a risk that can be minimized by preventive and therapeutic maneuvers.

  The patient with diabetes should have aggressive preventive dental services including frequent recall examinations, oral hygiene instructions, prophylaxis and treatment of periodontal disease.

  The diabetic patient should also be considered for antibiotics at a lower threshold than non-diabetics.

3. Dental management of patients with diabetes mellitus: specific guidelines

Based upon the HbA1c, one can determine the best protocol for dental management.

- **Patients under reasonable control (HbA1c <8.5)**

  In general, patients with HbA1c of less than 8.5 can be considered to be under fair control and dental management can follow normal dental protocol **(Table 20.2).**

  Consideration should be given to use of stress reduction protocol with oral conscious sedation or nitrous oxide.

  One should also have a low threshold to prescribe antibiotics in instances of concerns over odontogenic infections.

  Whenever there is a concern about management of diabetes through the dental intervention, medical consultations should be requested.

TABLE 20.2 Dental protocol for patients with adequate control

Time of appointment	Morning appointment
Diet	Normal breakfast; protect oral intake
Stress reduction	Patient rapport; short appointments (less than 3 hours)
Sedation protocol	Consider oral conscious sedation Consider use of nitrous oxide
All non-surgical and simple surgical procedures	Normal protocol Continue oral hypoglycemics or insulin
Complex prosthetic and surgical procedures	Consider sedation protocol Continue oral hypoglycemics or insulin For lengthy procedures, consult MD for changes in doses of hypoglycemics or insulin
Infection	Aggressive treatment of infection
Preventive protocol	More frequent recalls

- **Patients with poor diabetic control (HbA1c >8.5)** (Table 20.3)

  For patients with HbA1c of greater than 8.5, simple restorative and surgical procedures can be done under monitored environment.

  Complex elective surgery and restorative surgery should be deferred. The patient will have significant problems with healing and will have markedly increased risk for infection. These patients should have elective procedures deferred until their diabetes is under better control.

  When appropriate, sedation options such as oral conscious sedation or nitrous oxide should be considered.

TABLE 20.3 Dental management of diabetics with poor control (HbA1c >8.5)

Morning appointment with normal breakfast (less than 3 hours)
Continue oral hypoglycemics or insulin
Simple restorative and surgical procedures under monitored environment
Complex surgical and restorative procedures should be deferred
Stress reduction and sedation

21

DENTAL EVALUATION AND MANAGEMENT OF PATIENTS ON SEMAGLUTIDE AND TIRZEPATIDE (OZEMPIC, WEGOVY, MOUNJARO AND ZEPBOUND)

INTRODUCTION

Semaglutides and tirzepatides are increasingly used in patients with type 2 diabetes mellitus because of their effect on insulin production and amelioration of insulin resistance. More importantly, patients on these agents have a sense of satiety and decreased gastric emptying. This results in significant weight loss.

In fact, semaglutides and tirzepatides are now approved both for management of type 2 diabetes mellitus and for management of weight excess.

The dental practitioner will need to be mindful of the implications of these drugs on dentistry, particularly in relationship to dental surgery.

1. GLP-1 and GIP-1 receptor agonists

There has been a lot of information about how gut hormones are important in the regulation of metabolic processes. These gut hormones are called Incretins and are produced by cells lining the intestinal tract. Two gut hormones are particularly important.

- **Glucagon-like peptide-1 (GLP-1)**

  These are produced by the L cells in the lining of the intestinal tract. GLP-1 has a large number of functions **(Figure 21.1):**
  - Increases insulin production from the pancreas.
  - Decreases glucagon production from the pancreas.
  - Decreases peripheral resistance to insulin.
  - Acts on the brain to produce sense of satiety.
  - Acts on the brain to decrease appetite.

- Acts on the gastrointestinal tract to decrease gastrointestinal motility and decrease gastric emptying.
- Acts on the liver to decrease fat deposition in the liver.
- Acts on the liver to decrease lipid content in the liver.
- Beneficial effects on fatty liver (hepatic steatosis).

GLP-1 is therefore responsible for glucose homeostasis and regulation of appetite. These beneficial effects make this hormone an important therapeutic target. Currently a large number of GLP-1 receptor agonists are available therapeutically **(Table 21.1).** Among these, semaglutide is the most highly profiled receptor agonist because of its duration of action. Semaglutide is administered subcutaneously by the patient once a week. The dose of Semaglutide is gradually titrated up until the desired effect is accomplished.

- **Semaglutide (Ozempic and Wegovy)**
  For patients with type 2 diabetes mellitus, semaglutide is marketed as Ozempic. Semaglutide is also FDA-approved for weight loss and is marketed as Wegovy.

FIGURE 21.1 Glucagon-like peptide-1 (GLP-1)

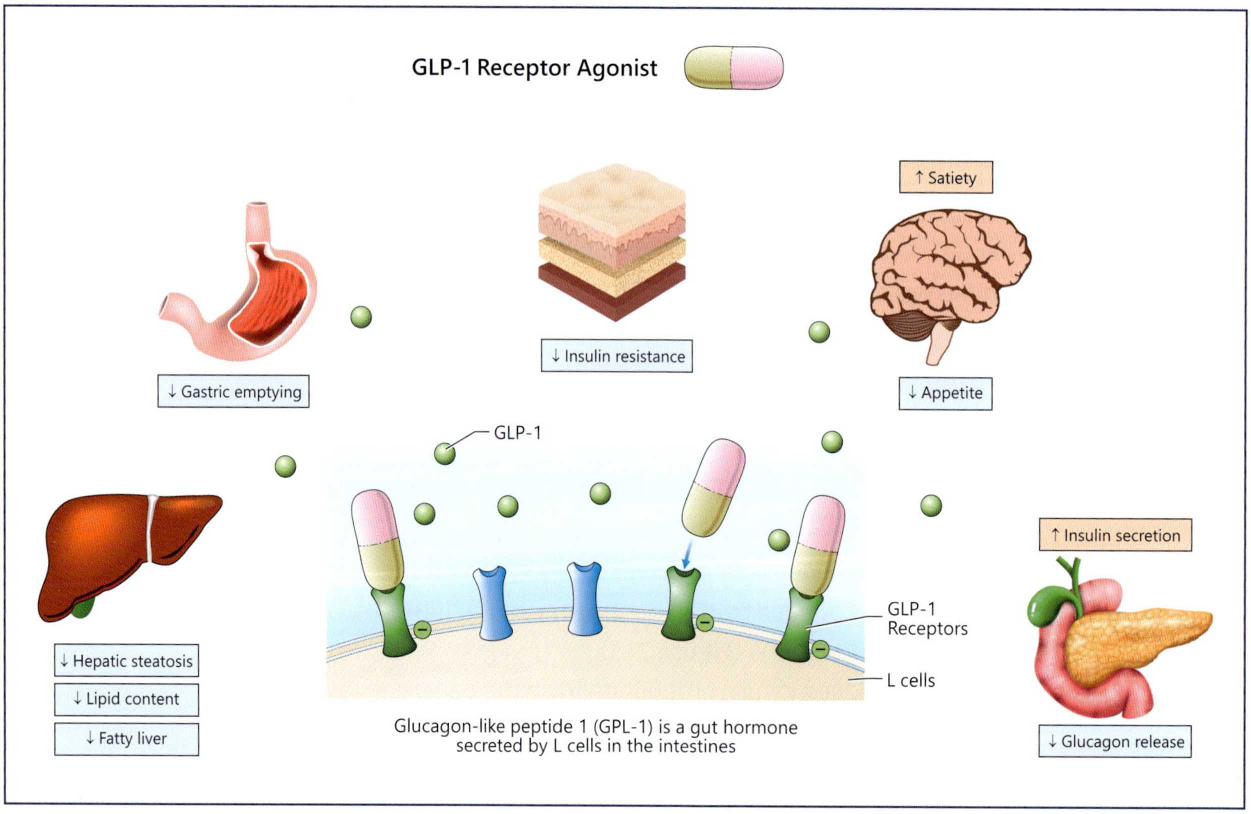

TABLE 21.1 Glucagon-like peptide-1 based therapy

Generic	Brand	Method of administration	FDA approved for weight loss
Dulaglutide	Trulicity	Weekly injections	No
Exenatide	Bydureon Beise	Weekly injections	No
Liraglutide	Victoza	Daily injections	No
Liraglutide	Liraglutide	Daily injections	Yes
Semaglutide	Ozempic	Weekly injections	No
Semaglutide	Rybelsus	Daily oral	No
Semaglutide	Wegovy	Daily injections	Yes

- **Gastric inhibitory polypeptide (GIP)**

  These are produced by the M cells in the lining of the intestinal tract. GIP has a large number of functions (**Figure 21.2**):

  - Increases insulin production from the pancreas.
  - Acts on the brain to produce sense of satiety.
  - Acts on the brain to decrease appetite.

FIGURE 21.2 Gastric inhibitory polypeptide (GIP)

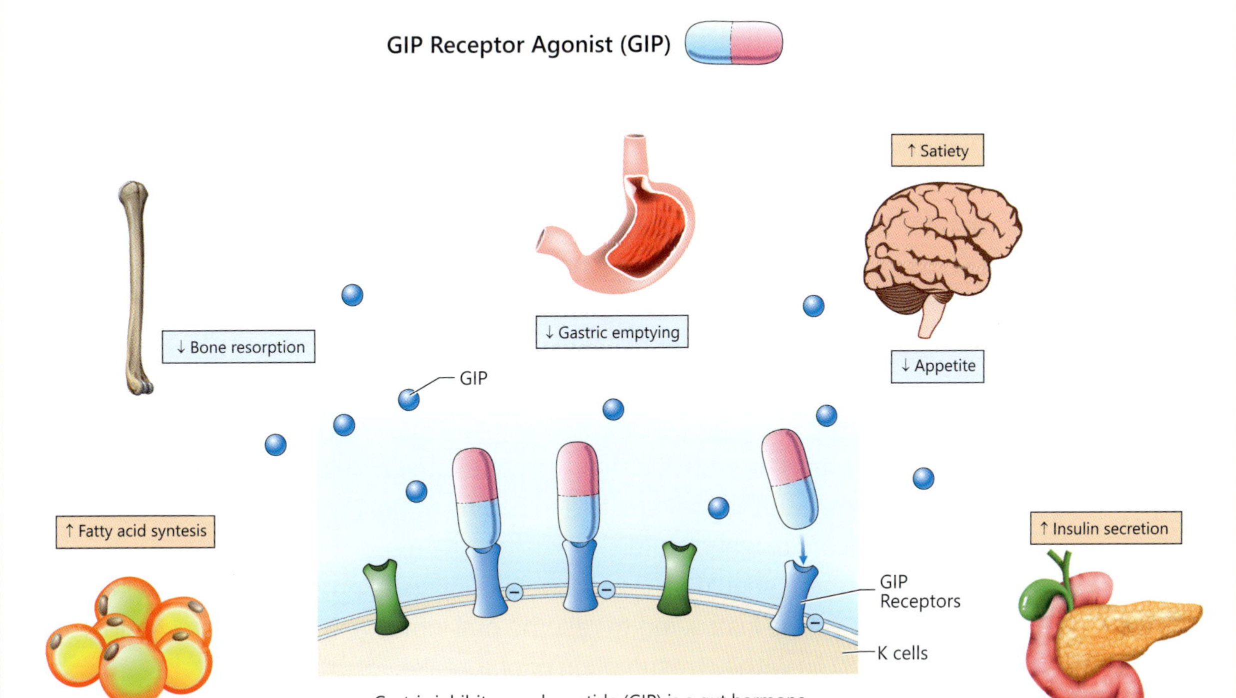

Gastric inhibitory polypeptide (GIP) is a gut hormone secreted by K cells in the intestines

- Acts on the gastrointestinal tract to decrease gastrointestinal motility and decrease gastric emptying.
- Acts on bone to decrease bone resorption.
- Increase fatty acid synthesis.

- **Tirzepatide (Mounjaro and Zepbound)**

  Tirzepatide is a dual target receptor agonist for both the L and the K cells and will produce both GLP-1 and GIP effects.

  In general, patients are on Mounjaro for management of type 2 diabetes mellitus. Zepbound is FDA approved version of the same drug for weight loss **(Table 21.2)**.

TABLE 21.2 Dual target glucagon-like peptide-1 and gastric inhibitory polypeptide based therapy

Generic	Brand	Method of administration	FDA approved for weight loss
Tirzepatide	Mounjaro	Weekly injections	No
Tirzepatide	Zepbound	Weekly injections	Yes

2. Dental evaluation of patients on GLP-1 and GIP receptor agonists

It is important to determine the indication for semaglutide and tirzepatide use. The protocol for the diabetic patient is slightly different than the patient with weight excess.

It is important to determine the medication that the patient is on, the dose of the medication and the timing of the administration of the medication.

3. Dental management of patients on GLP-1 and GIP receptor agonists

- **Diabetic patients**

  For the diabetic patient on semaglutide or tirzepatide, we need to **hold the medication for the week prior to planned dental surgery**. This is to minimize the likelihood of excessive gastroparesis at the time of dental intervention. The goal is to minimize the likelihood of aspiration during the procedure **(Table 21.3)**.

  The patient should be given the first morning appointment and be instructed to be NPO after midnight the night before.

  On the morning of the procedure, neither insulin nor oral hypoglycemic agents should be administered. It is probable that the patient might become hyperglycemic during the procedure, but this is preferable to having to deal with hypoglycemia in view of the NPO after midnight dictum.

  The appointment should be less than 3 hours so as not to run into the lunch hour. The patient will be instructed to resume oral intake and resume oral hypoglycemic agents or insulin with full resumption of oral intake.

TABLE 21.3 Dental protocol for diabetic patients on semaglutide or tirzepatide

Medication change	Hold semaglutide or tirzepatide for the week before the planned dental surgery
Time of appointment	Morning appointment
Diet	NPO after midnight; no breakfast
Stress reduction	Patient rapport; short appointments (less than 3 hours)
Sedation protocol	Consider oral conscious sedation Consider use of nitrous oxide
All non-surgical and simple surgical procedures	Normal protocol Hold oral hypoglycemics or insulin
Complex prosthetic and surgical procedures	Consider sedation protocol Hold oral hypoglycemics or insulin For lengthy procedures, consult MD
Infection	Aggressive treatment of infection
Preventive protocol	More frequent recalls

- **Patients on semaglutide or Mounjaro for weight management**

  For the patient on semaglutide or tirzepatide for weight management, we need to hold the medication for the week prior to planned dental surgery. This is to minimize the likelihood of excessive gastroparesis at the time of dental intervention. The goal is to minimize the likelihood of aspiration during the procedure (Table 21.4).

  The patient should be NPO after midnight so as to minimize the likelihood of aspiration. Semaglutide and tirzepatide can be resumed after the procedure.

TABLE 21.4 Dental protocol for patients on semaglutide or tirzepatide for weight management

Medication change	Hold semaglutide or tirzepatide for the week before the planned dental surgery
Time of appointment	Morning appointment
Diet	NPO after midnight; no breakfast
Stress reduction	Patient rapport; short appointments (less than 3 hours)
Sedation protocol	Consider oral conscious sedation Consider use of nitrous oxide
All non-surgical and simple surgical procedures	Normal protocol
Complex prosthetic and surgical procedures	Consider sedation protocol For lengthy procedures, consult MD

- **Patients on semaglutide or Mounjaro who is undertaking sedation dentistry**
  For the patient on semaglutide or tirzepatide who would need sedation dentistry, we need to **hold the medication for the week prior to planned dental surgery**. This is to minimize the likelihood of excessive gastroparesis at the time of dental intervention. The goal is to minimize the likelihood of aspiration during the procedure.
  The patient should be NPO after midnight and should hold all non-essential medications on the morning of sedation. In general, the clinician should start with low doses of the sedation drugs, IV or PO, and titrate up.

Increasing numbers of patients presenting to the dental practice will be on semaglutide or tirzepatide. It is important for the dental professional to understand the implications of these drugs on dental interventions.

22 DENTAL EVALUATION AND MANAGEMENT OF PATIENTS WITH THYROID DISEASE

INTRODUCTION

Thyroid disorders are common, and many patients are on medications for these conditions. It is important to understand the type of thyroid disorders the patient has, the medications they are on, the clinical status of the thyroid disorder and how they may impact dental management.

1. Dental evaluation of patients with thyroid diseases

A detailed medical history will help define if the thyroid disease will pose a problem for dental management. Fortunately, most patients with thyroid diseases are under adequate medical control and dental interventions can proceed without changes in protocol.

- **Hypothyroidism**
  Underactive thyroid is the most common thyroid disorder. The majority of patients with hypothyroidism have an autoimmune disorder called Hashimoto's thyroiditis. Hypothyroidism can also be the result of radioactive iodine therapy or surgical thyroidectomy.
  Patients are generally managed on various preparations of thyroid replacement, with synthetic thyroid (Synthroid) being the most commonly prescribed replacement therapy.

- **Hyperthyroidism**
  Overactive thyroid is less common and patients can be on anti-thyroid drugs such as methimazole or propylthiouracil. Patients with hyperthyroidism can also be on beta blockers for control of tachycardia.

Patients with hyperthyroidism might also be managed with radioactive iodine treatment or thyroidectomy. These patients often develop hypothyroidism after treatment.

- **Adequacy of control**
  Thyroid function is closely monitored by blood tests. Thyroid stimulating hormone (TSH) is an extremely sensitive way of monitoring thyroid function.

Understanding the type of thyroid disease the patient has and the adequacy of control will help with dental management of these patients.

2. Dental management of patients with thyroid diseases

In general, no changes in dental management are necessary if the patient's thyroid function is under good control.
Elective dental interventions should be deferred in patients whose thyroid function is not under good control.

- **Hypothyroidism**
  Patients with clinical hypothyroidism can have xerostomia, gingival disease and delayed healing. They may be more sensitive to vasoconstrictors in local anesthetics.

- **Hyperthyroidism**
  Patients with hyperthyroidism can have increased tooth decay, gingival disease and increased bone loss. They may be more sensitive to vasoconstrictors in local anesthetics.

3. Special concerns about analgesics and narcotics

Alteration in thyroid function can affect use of analgesics and narcotics.

- **Hypothyroidism**
  Patients with hypothyroidism may have blunted response to analgesics and narcotics. They also have slower metabolism and medications should be carefully titrated.

- **Hyperthyroidism**
  Patients with hyperthyroidism have a hyperdynamic cardiovascular system. Vasoconstrictors in these patients can induce tachycardia and hypertension.

In patients with thyroid diseases, attention should be given to the adequacy of control of the thyroid disease. When the thyroid function is in good range, dental procedures can proceed without changes in protocol. If the thyroid function is not adequately controlled, elective dental procedures should be delayed until thyroid function is normalized.

23

DENTAL EVALUATION AND MANAGEMENT OF THE PATIENT WITH ASTHMA

INTRODUCTION

Asthma is a common respiratory illness affecting children, adolescents and adults. Asthma is a reversible airway disease characterized by inflammation and narrowing of the airways, leading to symptoms such as wheezing, coughing or shortness of breath. It can be triggered by various factors such as allergens, exercise, cold air, respiratory infections and stress. The goal is to avoid elective dental interventions in patients not under ideal control such as to minimize the likelihood of acute exacerbation in the dental chair.

1. Medical evaluation of patients with asthma

Asthma is characterized according to severity of disease. Understanding the specific categories will allow the dental professional to assess severity of disease and the likelihood of acute exacerbations.

- **Intermittent**
    - Symptoms occurring two or fewer days per week.
    - Use of short-acting beta agonist to relieve symptoms two or fewer times a week.
    - No interference with normal activities between exacerbations.
    - Pulmonary function tests in normal range between exacerbations.
    - Rare exacerbations requiring oral glucocorticoids.

- **Mild persistent**
    - Symptoms more than twice weekly though less than daily.
    - Use of short-acting beta agonist to relieve symptoms more than twice weekly (but not daily).

- Minor interference with normal activities.
- Two or more exacerbations per year requiring oral glucocorticoids.

- **Moderate persistent**
  - Daily symptoms.
  - Daily need of reliever therapy for symptom relief.
  - Some limitation of normal activity.
  - Compromise of pulmonary function tests.

- **Severe**
  - Presence of symptoms throughout the day.
  - Need for reliever therapy several times a day.
  - Significant limitation of activity.
  - Need for emergency room intervention or hospitalization.

While each category has distinctive features that mandate different treatment, the goal is to optimize control and avoid exacerbations. The dental professional should be familiar with the clinical features and the therapeutic options for any patient presenting with varying severity of disease.

2. Medical management of the patient with asthma

Regardless of the severity of disease, the goal of medical therapy is to optimize the degree of control. The different medications used for control of asthma are listed in Table 23.1. Medical management of asthma is often in steps dictated by the severity of disease:

- **Intermittent (Step 1)**
  - Avoid triggers that can precipitate an acute exacerbation.
  - Use of short-acting beta agonist for symptom relief.
  - Combination of low-dose inhaled glucocorticoids with a fast-acting long-acting beta agonist such as busenolide-formeterol.

- **Mild persistent (Step 2)**
  - Daily low-dose inhaled glucocorticoid.
  - Use of short-acting beta agonist for symptomatic relief.
  - Use of leukotriene modifiers as an alternative.

- **Moderate persistent (Step 3)**
  - Daily low-dose inhaled glucocorticoid and long-acting beta agonist.
  - Use of inhaled glucocorticoid and short-acting beta agonist for acute symptoms.
  - Addition of long-acting muscarinic antagonist.
  - Use of leukotriene modifier.

- **Severe persistent (Steps 4 and 5)**
  - Medium or high dose inhaled glucocorticoid in combination with a long-acting beta glucocorticoid.
  - Long-acting muscarinic antagonist.
  - Leukotriene modifier.
  - Daily or alternate day steroids.
  - Immunomodifier with targeted monoclonal antibodies.

For the dental professional, the type of medications the patient is on will provide a good assessment of the severity of disease and a meaningful way to risk stratify the patient.

TABLE 23.1 Commonly used medications for management of asthma

Commonly prescribed medications	
Inhalant	**Steroid inhalant** Fluticasone proprionate (Flovent) Budesonide (Pulmicort) Flunisolide (Aerobid) Triamcinolone acetonide (Azmacort) Fluticasone furoate (Ellipta) Ciclesonide (Alvesco) Mometasone furoate (Asmanex) **Short-acting beta-2 agonists** Salbutamol (Albuterol, Proventil, Ventolin) Metaproterenol (Alupent, Metaprel) Terbutaline (Brethine) Pinbuterol (Maxair) **Long-acting beta-2 agonists** Salmeterol (Serevent) Formoterol (Foradil) **Long-acting muscarinic antagonists** Ipratropium (Atrovent) Tiotropium (Spiriva) **Combination steroid/beta-2 agonists** Fluticasone/Salmeterol (Advair) Budesonide/Formoterol (Symbicort) **Combination steroid/anticholinergic agent/beta-2 agonists** Fluticasone/Umeclidinium/Vilanterol (Trelegy)
Leukotriene antagonists	Montelukast (Singulair) Zafirlukast (Accolate) Zileuton (Zyflo)

Commonly prescribed medications	
Mast cell stabilizers	Cromoglicate (Cromylyn) Nedocromil (Tilade)
Steroids	Prednisone
Immunomodulators	Omalizumab Mepolizumab Reslizumab Benaralizumab

Regardless of the severity of the disease, the goal is to optimize control of the disease and prevent exacerbations.

3. Dental evaluation of the patient with asthma

Careful evaluation of the severity of disease, the medications the patient is on and the current adequacy of control of disease is important for the dental management of the patient with asthma. The goal is to avoid an acute exacerbation of respiratory symptoms in the dental chair.

- **Medical history**

  Although patients may have different disease severity, the dental evaluation should concentrate on the stability of the patient's respiratory symptoms.
  The list of medications the patient is on will also tell you about the severity of disease.
  Record the triggers of asthmatic attacks, particularly stress, which may be encountered during a dental procedure.
  It would be important to ask if the patient has had prior acute exacerbations during dental procedures.

- **Medications the patient is on for asthma**

  All medications the patient is on for asthma should be reviewed. Note should be taken for patients on beta agonists and steroids as it will affect dental management.

- **Sedation dentistry**

  Patients with asthma seek sedation dentistry as it would minimize stress as a trigger for acute exacerbation. Careful evaluation of the stability of the patient's disease would permit optimal selection of the patient most suited to sedation dentistry (Chapter 45).

4. Dental management of the patient with asthma

- **Adequacy of control**

  Elective dentistry should be avoided in all patients with marginal control of asthma. The likelihood of acute exacerbation during the dental procedure is high in these patients.

- **Timing of dental procedures**
  The patient should be scheduled for the first appointment of the day, at which time the endogenous catecholamines would be at the highest level.
  The appointments should be short (less than 3 hours) to minimize stress.

- **Medications the patient is on for asthma**
  The patient should be instructed to take all of their morning medications on the day of the procedure.
  The patient should specifically be reminded to bring the specific short-term reliever inhaler to the appointment on the off chance that an acute exacerbation occurs.

- **Local anesthetic with vasoconstrictors**
  Since the patient is usually already on a short-acting or long-acting beta agonist, local anesthetics with vasoconstrictors should be restricted to 2 carpules of 1:100,000 epinephrine or 1:50,000 levonordefrin.

- **Post-operative pain control**
  Unless the patient is on systemic glucocorticoids, analgesics, non-steroidal anti-inflammatory drugs and narcotics can be administered safely.
  In patients on systemic glucocorticoids, non-steroidal anti-inflammatory drugs should be avoided.

- **Infection**
  Patients on inhaled or systemic glucocorticoids or immunomodulators are at increased risk of infection. Judicious use of antibiotics may be necessary.

- **Wound healing**
  Patients on inhaled or systemic glucocorticoids or immunomodulators may have increased issues with wound healing.

- **Sedation dentistry**
  Sedation dentistry can be offered to patients with good control of their symptoms (Chapter 43).

Although management of patients with chronic asthma can be quite complicated, the dental professional should lean heavily on the adequacy of control for evaluation and management of patients for optimal care. The goal is to exclude patients with inadequate control to elective dental procedure so as not to have to address acute exacerbation of asthma. The patient should be carefully instructed to bring the short-relief inhaler to the dental appointment.

24 DENTAL EVALUATION AND MANAGEMENT OF THE PATIENT WITH CHRONIC OBSTRUCTIVE PULMONARY DISEASE

INTRODUCTION

Chronic obstructive pulmonary disease is a common respiratory illness characterized by cough, shortness of breath and airflow limitation. Medical management revolves around decreasing shortness of breath and reducing the frequency of acute exacerbations. Dental evaluation and management should revolve around performing procedures only when the clinical situation is stable in order to avoid acute exacerbation.

1. Medical evaluation of patients with chronic obstructive pulmonary disease

There is considerable overlap of several closely related common respiratory diseases: Chronic obstructive pulmonary disease, chronic bronchitis, emphysema and chronic obstructive pulmonary disease. Chronic obstructive pulmonary disease is defined as a heterogenous lung condition characterized by chronic respiratory symptoms (cough, shortness of breath, sputum production) due to abnormalities of the airway and/or alveoli.

- **Chronic bronchitis**
    - Chronic productive cough over an extended period.
    - Symptoms of at least 3 months over each of successive 2 years.
    - Intermittent exacerbations.

- **Emphysema**
    - Enlargement of airspaces distal to the terminal bronchioles.
    - Destruction of airspace walls.
    - Significant airflow limitations.
    - Intermittent exacerbations.

- **Chronic obstructive pulmonary disease**
    - Reversible airway obstruction.
    - Clinical features and management covered in previous chapter.

While each condition has distinctive features that mandate different treatment, there is significant overlap in these conditions, necessitating specific treatment for any given individual. The dental professional should be familiar with the clinical features and the therapeutic options for any patient presenting with the diagnosis of chronic obstructive pulmonary disease.

2. Medical management of the patient with chronic obstructive pulmonary disease

Regardless of the severity of disease, the goal of medical therapy is to optimize degree of control.

Smoking cessation is critical for all patients.

Different medication regimens would be designed to optimize respiratory function of patients with chronic obstructive pulmonary disease. Medications may include **(Table 24.1):**

- Short-acting beta agonists.
- Long-acting beta agonists.
- Inhaled steroids.
- Long-acting muscarinic antagonists.
- Combinations drugs.
- Systemic glucocorticoids.

Multiple medications may be required for symptom management of the patient. Attempts are made to come to a medication combination that would prevent acute exacerbations. Not infrequently, this would include a short-acting beta agonist for acute exacerbations. For maintenance, long-acting beta agonists, long-acting muscarinic antagonists and inhaled glucocorticoids are often used in different combinations. In instances of severe chronic obstructive pulmonary disease, systemic steroids or supplemental oxygen may be necessary.

TABLE 24.1 Commonly used medications for management of chronic obstructive pulmonary disease

Commonly prescribed medications	
Inhalant	**Steroid inhalant** Fluticasone proprionate (Flovent) Budesonide (Pulmicort) Flunisolide (Aerobid) Triamcinolone acetonide (Azmacort) Fluticasone furoate (Ellipta) Ciclesonide (Alvesco) Mometasone furoate (Asmanex) **Short-acting beta-2 agonists** Salbutamol (Albuterol, Proventil, Ventolin) Metaproterenol (Alupent, Metaprel) Terbutaline (Brethine) Pinbuterol (Maxair) **Long-acting beta-2 agonists** Salmeterol (Serevent) Formoterol (Foradil) **Long-acting muscarinic antagonists** Ipratropium (Atrovent) Tiotropium (Spiriva) **Combination steroid/beta-2 agonists** Fluticasone/Salmeterol (Advair) Budesonide/Formoterol (Symbicort) **Combination steroid/anticholinergic agent/beta-2 agonists** Fluticasone/Umeclidinium/Vilanterol (Trelegy)
Steroids	Prednisone
Oxygen supplementation	Low flow oxygen chronically

3. Dental evaluation of the patient with chronic obstructive pulmonary disease

Careful evaluation of the severity of disease, the medications the patient is on and the current adequacy of control of disease is important for the dental management of the patient with chronic obstructive pulmonary disease. The goal is to avoid an acute exacerbation of respiratory symptoms in the dental chair.

- **Medical history**

  Although the exact contribution of the various overlapping syndromes of chronic obstructive pulmonary disease, chronic bronchitis, emphysema and chronic obstructive pulmonary disease may be difficult, the dental evaluation should concentrate on the stability of the patient's respiratory symptoms.

  The list of medications the patient is on will also tell you about the severity of disease. Record the triggers of chronic obstructive pulmonary disease attacks, particularly stress, which may be encountered during a dental procedure.

  It would be important to ask if the patient has had prior acute exacerbations during dental procedures.

- **Medications the patient is on for chronic obstructive pulmonary disease**

  All medications the patient is on for chronic obstructive pulmonary disease should be reviewed. Note should be taken for patients on beta agonists and steroids as it will affect dental management.

- **Sedation dentistry**

  Patients with chronic obstructive pulmonary disease may seek sedation dentistry as it would minimize stress as a trigger for acute exacerbation. However, it is critical to understand that some patients have issues with CO_2 retention. Sedation in this setting can markedly accentuate hypercarbia and precipitate respiratory arrest. Prior to any consideration of sedation, consultation with the patient's pulmonologist is essential to assess prior history of CO_2 retention. No patients with history of retention should be offered sedation dentistry.

4. Dental management of the patient with chronic obstructive pulmonary disease

- **Adequacy of control**

  Elective dentistry should be avoided in all patients with marginal control of chronic obstructive pulmonary disease. The likelihood of acute exacerbation during the dental procedure is high in these patients.

- **Timing of dental procedures**

  The patient should be scheduled for the first appointment of the day, at which time the endogenous catecholamines would be at the highest level.

  The appointments should be short (less than 3 hours) to minimize stress.

- **Medications the patient is on for chronic obstructive pulmonary disease**

  The patient should be instructed to take all of their morning medications on the day of the procedure.

  The patient should specifically be reminded to bring the specific short-term reliever inhaler to the appointment on the off chance that we encounter an acute exacerbation.

- **Local anesthetic with vasoconstrictors**
  Since the patient is usually already on short-acting or long-acting beta agonist, local anesthetics with vasoconstrictors should be restricted to 2 carpules of 1:100,000 epinephrine or 1:50,000 levonordefrin.

- **Post-operative pain control**
  Unless the patient is on systemic glucocorticoids, analgesics, non-steroidal anti-inflammatory drugs and narcotics can be administered safely.
  In patients on systemic glucocorticoids, non-steroidal anti-inflammatory drugs should be avoided.

- **Infection**
  Patients on inhaled or systemic glucocorticoids or immunomodulators are at increased risk of infection. Judicious use of antibiotics may be necessary.

- **Wound healing**
  Patients on inhaled or systemic glucocorticoids or immunomodulators may have increased issues with wound healing.

- **Sedation dentistry**
  Patients with chronic obstructive pulmonary disease may seek sedation dentistry as it would minimize stress as a trigger for acute exacerbation. Sedation dentistry should not be offered to patients with resting hypoxemia or history of CO_2 retention (Chapter 45).

Although management of the patient with chronic obstructive pulmonary disease can be quite complicated, the dental professional should lean heavily on the adequacy of control for evaluation and management of patient for optimal care. The goal is to exclude patients with inadequate control to elective dental procedure so as not to have to address acute exacerbation of chronic obstructive pulmonary disease. The patient should be carefully instructed to bring the short-relief inhaler to the dental appointment.

25 DENTAL EVALUATION AND MANAGEMENT OF THE PATIENT WITH HEPATITIS

INTRODUCTION

Inflammatory and infectious diseases of the liver can complicate dental management of the patient. Hepatitis can be the result of a whole array of viruses or the result of toxins such as alcohol and drugs. It is important to understand the cause of the hepatitis, the current status of the disease in order to adjust dental management of the patient.

1. Dental evaluation of patients with hepatitis

A detailed medical history will help define the cause of hepatitis and the treatment.

- **Hepatitis A**

  Hepatitis A is a mild viral infection, usually spread through contaminated food and water or through close contact. It is a self-limited disease, and patients generally recover within a few weeks.

- **Acute hepatitis B**

  Hepatitis B is a viral infection that is usually spread through contact with infected blood or bodily fluids, such as semen or vaginal secretions. Patients can have mild to severe disease and can have resultant liver damage.

  During active infection, patients have hepatitis B antigen in the blood stream and are infective.

  Acute hepatitis B is generally a self-limited disease and resolves without serious hepatic sequelae. Patients are managed with supportive care.

  In some instances of serious disease, antivirals may be used.

- **Chronic hepatitis B**

  A small portion of patients with hepatitis B fail to clear the virus and have chronic antigenemia. These patients are infective and can have progression of disease to cirrhosis.

  These patients are followed with serial liver enzyme determinations, Fibroscan to determine extent of fibrosis of the liver, liver biopsy to assess status of infection and hepatitis B DNA titer.

  Patients are often treated with antivirals such as tenofovir, entecavir, lamivudine, telbivudine or adefovir.

- **Hepatitis C**

  Hepatitis C is a chronic infection usually spread through contact with infected blood or body fluids. Patients are often asymptomatic but have fluctuating liver function tests. Untreated, patients with hepatitis C can progress to develop cirrhosis.

  Fifteen percent of patients have a self-limited disease with no sequelae.

  Eighty-five percent of patients with hepatitis C do not clear the virus and would be candidates for treatment with combinations of direct-acting antivirals (DAA) such as sofobuvir, ledipasvir, daclatasvir and flecaprevir/pibrentasvir. Choice of antiviral is dependent upon the genotype of hepatitis C. With completion of treatment, the patient would be cleared of hepatitis C.

  Decision to treat is dependent upon hepatitis C viral load by DNA titer, extent of liver function test abnormalities, genotype of the virus and extent of fibrosis by Fibroscan.

- **Non-alcoholic steatohepatitis (NASH) or fatty liver**

  Non-alcoholic steatohepatitis (NASH) is the result of accumulation of fat in the liver, causing inflammation and damage to the liver cells. Although the disease progresses slowly, it can result in cirrhosis. NASH is associated with obesity, type 2 diabetes mellitus and high cholesterol.

  Treatment is directed against management of weight excess, type 2 diabetes and hyperlipidemia.

  NASH is becoming an increasingly common cause of cirrhosis and should be carefully identified, evaluated and managed in order not to interfere with planned dental interventions.

- **Alcoholic hepatitis**

  Alcoholic hepatitis is the result of heavy and prolonged use of alcohol. Treatment is dependent upon early identification of the problem and emphasizes complete abstinence. Left untreated, it can progress to cirrhosis.

- **Drug induced hepatitis**
  Rarely, prolonged exposures to medications can result in inflammation of the liver. Left untreated, this can progress to liver failure. Treatment is predicated upon the correct identification and cessation of the offending agent.

Understanding the type of hepatitis the patient has and the treatment they are on will help with dental management of these patients.

2. Dental management of the patient with hepatitis

Proper dental management of the patients with hepatitis is dependent upon the current status of the hepatitis and the current liver function.
In general, one should avoid elective dentistry in the setting of active hepatitis.
The liver is responsible for synthesis of a large number of proteins. The key proteins of dental relevance are the coagulation factors. In instances where there is compromise of synthesis of the hepatic coagulation factors (Factors II, VII and IX and X), there is an increased risk of bleeding.
The liver is also responsible for detoxification and metabolism of a many drugs. In instances of hepatic compromise, many of the drugs used in dentistry will need to be modified, if not completely avoided.
Elective dental interventions should be deferred in patients with active disease or changing liver function tests.
Dental management is also predicated upon the type of hepatitis the patient has.

- **Hepatitis A**
  Most patients with hepatitis A have a mild and self-limited disease that resolve without sequelae.
  In patients with active hepatitis A infection, elective dental procedures should be deferred. Otherwise, one can proceed with normal protocol.

- **Acute hepatitis B**
  Patients with an acute episode of hepatitis B have active viral replications and changing liver function tests. All procedures should be deferred until the patient has recovered from the infection.
  After recovery, the patient would have antibodies to hepatitis B and would have cleared the hepatitis B antigen. Liver function tests usually return to normal and the patient can be treated with normal protocols.

- **Chronic hepatitis B**
  Patients with chronic hepatitis B have persistent antigenemia, are infective and may have fluctuating liver function tests. Patients may be on antiviral therapy.

If the liver function tests indicate no synthetic abnormalities (normal PT/INR as a reflection of adequate production of coagulation factors) and no detoxification issues, dentistry can proceed with normal protocol with attention to hemostasis.
Acetaminophen has to be used judiciously with a maximal daily dose not to exceed 1,500 mg.
Drugs that are hepatically metabolized should be used judiciously.

- **Hepatitis C**

  Patients with hepatitis C that have been treated successfully with antiviral therapy, have negative hepatitis C DNA titers, have normal synthetic and detoxification function can be managed with normal protocol.
  Those that have not been treated have to be carefully assessed with respect to the liver function tests and elective procedures should be deferred until hepatitis C is successfully treated.
  Acetaminophen has to be used judiciously with a maximal daily dose not to exceed 1,500 mg.
  Drugs that are hepatically metabolized should be used judiciously.

- **Non-alcoholic steatohepatitis (NASH) or fatty liver**

  In general, these patients have mild synthetic and detoxification compromises and can be managed with careful attention to hemostasis.
  Acetaminophen has to be used judiciously with a maximal daily dose not to exceed 1,500 mg.
  Drugs that are hepatically metabolized should be used judiciously.

- **Alcoholic hepatitis**

  Dental management is largely predicated upon the extent of hepatic injury the patient has sustained.
  Significant issues with synthetic and detoxification function can be assessed through liver function tests and PT/INR. In instances where there is concern over adequate liver function, elective procedures should be deferred.
  In other instances, dental procedures should be done with careful attention to bleeding diathesis.
  Acetaminophen has to be used judiciously with a maximal daily dose not to exceed 1,500 mg.
  Drugs that are hepatically metabolized should be used judiciously.

- **Drug induced hepatitis**

  In general, the liver function tests return to normal after withdrawal of offending agents and dentistry can proceed using normal protocol.

In instances where there is concern over residual hepatic compromise, dental procedures should be done with careful attention to bleeding diathesis.
Acetaminophen has to be used judiciously with a maximal daily dose not to exceed 1,500 mg.
Drugs that are hepatically metabolized should be used judiciously.

3. Special concerns about analgesics, sedatives and narcotics

Alteration in liver function can affect use of analgesics, local anesthetics, sedatives and narcotics commonly prescribed in dentistry.

- **Acetaminophen**
  Acetaminophen should be avoided in patients with severe liver compromise.
  Otherwise, it has to be used judiciously with a maximal daily dose not to exceed 1,500 mg.

- **Aspirin**
  Aspirin is infrequently used in dentistry and should be avoided because of coagulation concerns and thrombocytopenia.

- **Non-steroidal anti-inflammatory drugs**
  All non-steroidal anti-inflammatory drugs should be avoided in view of concerns over coagulation, thrombocytopenia and bleeding disorder.

- **Sedatives**
  Almost all of the drugs used for sedation is metabolized by the liver via the CYP3A4 pathway. In instances of liver function compromise where sedation is deemed important, agents such as lorazepam which is not metabolized by the CYP3A4 enzyme system can be used judiciously. Sedation dentistry can be offered only to patients with sufficient hepatic reserve to metabolize medications administered (Chapter 45).

- **Narcotics**
  The liver is responsible for metabolizing and eliminating most of the narcotics used in dentistry. In instances of liver function impairment, this can result in accumulation of narcotics because of decreased metabolism.
  Most importantly, in patients with severe liver function compromise, narcotics can precipitate hepatic encephalopathy, a potentially lethal complication.
  Many of the narcotics used in dentistry are in combination with acetaminophen. Acetaminophen has to be used judiciously with a maximal daily dose not to exceed 1,500 mg.

In patients with a history of hepatitis, attention should be given to the current activity of the disease, the adequacy of liver function, the coagulation status and the platelet count prior to consideration of elective dental interventions.
PT/INR, platelet count, liver function tests and consultation with the patient's physician should be done prior to planned elective dental procedures.
During the procedure, care should be taken to minimize the use of local anesthetics and vasoconstrictors. Extra attention should be given to local hemostasis. Sedation should be avoided in patients with significant liver function compromise.
After the procedure, use of analgesics and narcotics should be carefully reviewed to avoid complications.

26 DENTAL EVALUATION AND MANAGEMENT OF THE PATIENT WITH CIRRHOSIS

INTRODUCTION

Cirrhosis of the liver can complicate dental management of the patient. Cirrhosis can be the result of a whole array etiologies, ranging from hepatitis, non-alcoholic steatohepatitis (NASH) or toxins such as alcohol and drugs. Patients with cirrhosis are at increased risk of bleeding, delayed healing and significant sensitivity to drugs commonly used for dentistry. It is important to consult the patient's physician prior to elective intervention.

1. Dental evaluation of patients with cirrhosis

A detailed medical history will help define the cause of cirrhosis, the current status of the liver and the treatment rendered to the patient to date.

- **Medical history**
  In consultation with the patient's physician, it is important to establish the cause of cirrhosis in the patient, and the extent of liver function derangement, with particular attention to any bleeding or clotting disorders. Attention should be given to the current overall functional status of the patient prior to planned elective dental intervention. Medications the patient is on should be carefully assessed with respect to implication for the dental procedures.

- **Assessment of coagulation disorders**
  Abnormality of the synthetic function of the liver can result in compromises of production of coagulation factors (Factors I, VII, IX, X in particular, Factors V, XI, XII, XIII to a lesser extent), which can accentuate bleeding disorders.

Cirrhosis can also result in hypersplenism, which in turn can cause issues with thrombocytopenia.
It is important to determine CBC and PT/INR prior to any elective dental interventions.

- **Assessment of liver function**
  The liver is also integral in the detoxification of drugs. A liver function panel is important to assess the ability of the liver to detoxify drugs commonly used in dentistry.

Careful assessment prior to dental interventions will optimize the success of dental intervention.

2. Dental management of the patient with cirrhosis

Proper dental management of the patients with cirrhosis is dependent upon the current status of the liver, the coagulation status, the platelet count and the current liver function.
In general, one should avoid elective dentistry in the setting of coagulation disorder (prolonged PT/INR and platelet count less than 50,000) or changing liver function tests since the risks are markedly increased.

- **Coagulation concerns**
  It would be prudent to defer elective dental intervention if the PT/INR is greater than 2 or if the platelet count is less than 50,000.
  Local hemostatic measures should be deployed to optimize hemostasis: extra sutures, compressive packing and dressings, use of microfibrillar collagen hemostat, oxidized cellulose, topical thrombin and tranexamic acid should all be considered.

- **Local anesthetics and Vasoconstrictors**
  Metabolism and elimination of local anesthetics can be compromised. As a result, the clearance of local anesthetics may be impaired. Care should be taken to minimize the dose of local anesthetics used.
  Impaired liver function can also result in decreased clearance of vasoconstrictors. It is important to limit the use of vasoconstrictors to 2 ampules of epinephrine at 1;100,000 and 2 ampules of levonordefrin at 1:50,000 at each session.

- **Antibiotics**
  Patients with cirrhosis often have compromised immunity and poor healing. Antibiotics may be necessary in their management. Certain antibiotics should be avoided in patients with cirrhosis: azithromycin, doxycycline, clindamycin and metronidazole should all be avoided or used judiciously.

3. Special concerns about analgesics, sedatives and narcotics

Alteration in liver function can affect use of analgesics, local anesthetics, sedatives and narcotics commonly prescribed in dentistry.

- **Acetaminophen**

  Acetaminophen should be avoided in patients with severe liver compromise. Otherwise, it has to be judiciously with a maximal daily dose not to exceed 1,500 mg.

- **Aspirin**

  Aspirin is infrequently used in dentistry and should be avoided because of coagulation concerns and thrombocytopenia.

- **Non-steroidal anti-inflammatory drugs**

  All non-steroidal anti-inflammatory drugs should be avoided in view of concerns over coagulation, thrombocytopenia and bleeding disorder.

- **Sedatives**

  Almost all of the drugs used for sedation are metabolized by the liver via the CYP3A4 pathway. In instances of liver function compromise where sedation is deemed important, agents such as lorazepam, which is not metabolized by the CYP3A4 enzyme system, can be used judiciously.

- **Narcotics**

  The liver is responsible for metabolizing and eliminating most of the narcotics used in dentistry. In instances of liver function impairment, this can result in accumulation of narcotics because of decreased metabolism.

  Most importantly, in patients with severe liver function compromise, narcotics can precipitate hepatic encephalopathy, a potentially lethal complication.

  Many of the narcotics used in dentistry are in combination with acetaminophen. Acetaminophen has to be used judiciously with a maximal daily dose not to exceed 1,500 mg.

In patients with cirrhosis, attention should be given to the current activity of the disease, the adequacy of liver function, the coagulation status and the platelet count prior to consideration of elective dental interventions.

PT/INR, platelet count, liver function tests and consultation with the patient's physician should be done prior to planned elective dental procedures.

During the procedure, care should be taken to minimize the use of local anesthetics and vasoconstrictors. Extra attention should be given to local hemostasis. Sedation should be avoided in patients with cirrhosis.

After the procedure, use of analgesics and narcotics should be limited to avoid complications.

27 DENTAL EVALUATION AND MANAGEMENT OF THE PATIENT WITH LIVER TRANSPLANT

INTRODUCTION

Liver transplant is the final option for patients with end stage liver disease. Although a child may be able to have a segment of liver donated from a living donor, the majority of the liver transplants are done with a cadaver donor. Waiting on the list for a suitable liver is often a long process, and the patient is often quite debilitated coming to the transplant.
All patients after liver transplantation will require life-long immunosuppression. They are usually on combinations of drugs working in different paths of immune response:

- Glucocorticoids.
- Antimetabolites such as mycophenolate, or less commonly, azathioprine.
- Calcineurin inhibitors such as tacrolimus, sirolimus or less commonly, cyclosporine.

Medications the patient is on after liver transplant may have oral complications and may require specific dental attention.
Different transplant programs have different protocols for antibiotic premedication for dental procedures. It is important for the dental professional to get medical clearance from the transplant team to accommodate the special needs of any given patient.
Patients with liver transplants are more prone to infections, including dental infections. It is important to have heightened attention to the patient's oral health and to use antibiotics for management of odontogenic infections.

1. Dental management of patients before liver transplant

In general, it is recommended that the patients do not undergo elective dental procedures for the first 6 months after transplant. It is therefore recommended that the dental health be optimized as much as possible prior to planned transplant.

- **Dental cleaning**
  It is important to have a thorough dental cleaning before the procedure to optimize oral health going into transplant.

- **Management of gingival disease**
  Gingival hyperplasia is a common complication of some of the immunosuppressive drugs. It is therefore important to treat gingival disease prior to transplant to minimize infection after the transplant.

- **Tooth extractions**
  Any problematic teeth that may cause infection should be extracted prior to transplant.

- **Oral hygiene instructions**
  The patient should be instructed on proper oral hygiene techniques to optimize oral health going into the transplant and after the transplant.

By addressing these oral health issues before the liver transplant, the patient should have fewer complications after the transplant when dental interventions would be significantly more complicated.

2. Dental management for the first 6 months after transplant

Except for extenuating circumstances, it is important to avoid elective dental procedures for the first 6 months after transplant. Immunosuppressive drugs tend to be at the highest level during this period, thereby interfering with wound healing and increasing the likelihood of infection.

In instances where dental procedures have to be done, it is important to consult the transplant team in order to assess the need for antibiotic premedication and post-operative antibiotics. It is important to discuss medications that may need to be prescribed peri-operatively in order to minimize the likelihood of drug-drug interactions.

3. Dental management of the patient after 6 months post-transplant

It is important to aggressively address oral health of the patient following liver transplant. The patients are more prone to oral infections, which can result in systemic infection that can greatly complicate the patient's welfare.

- **Oral hygiene instructions**
  The patient should be instructed on proper oral hygiene techniques to optimize oral health.

- **Dental cleaning**
  Frequent recalls are appropriate in these patients in order to optimize oral health.

- **Management of gingival disease**
  Gingival hyperplasia is a common complication of some of the immunosuppressive drugs, particularly cyclosporine.
  Meticulous home oral health care and frequent recalls will minimize this complication.

4. Dental implications of immunosuppressive drugs

Medications commonly prescribed after transplant can have important dental implication. In general, infections are more common on immunosuppressive drugs. It is also important to understand that medications the dental professional may prescribe can have drug-drug interactions with the immunosuppressive drugs and can interfere with their efficacy.
It is important to connect with the transplant team prior to elective interventions to coordinate the optimal management of the patient.

- **Steroids**
  Steroids are commonly prescribed after a transplant. The dose of steroids is weaned rapidly during the first months after transplant. Adrenal insufficiency is generally not an issue beyond the first 6 months after transplant and stress dose steroids are generally not necessary.
  However, steroids do impair healing and increase the likelihood of infection.
  It is important that you address these issues with the transplant team to be sure that there is no need for adjustment of the steroid dose.

- **Tacrolimus**
  Tacrolimus can cause mild gingival hyperplasia. It can also cause xerostomia. Both conditions can promote gingival inflammation, infection and tooth decay.

- **Sirolimus**
  Sirolimus can lead to oral ulcers, which need to be addressed with topical management.
  Sirolimus can also cause xerostomia, which can lead to infection and tooth decay.

- **Mycophenolate**
  Mycophenolate can cause xerostomia.

- **Cyclosporine**
  Cyclosporine can cause significant gingival hyperplasia. Fortunately, cyclosporine has been progressively phased out, yielding to the newer immunosuppressants.

5. Need for antibiotic premedication for dental procedures

There are no specific guidelines that are uniformly adopted. Different transplant centers have different protocols. It is therefore important to discuss the need for premedication with the transplant team prior to elective surgery.
If antibiotic premedication is deemed necessary, amoxicillin 2 g should be given an hour before planned procedure to patients without penicillin allergy (Table 27.1).
For patients with penicillin allergy, cephalexin 2 g should be given an hour before planned procedure. Cephalexin should not be used in patients with history of anaphylaxis, urticaria or angioedema to penicillin or ampicillin (Table 27.1).

TABLE 27.1 Antibiotics for premedication in liver transplant patients

Premedication given one hour before procedure	
No penicillin allergy	**Penicillin allergy**
Amoxicillin 2 g	Cephalexin 2 g Should not be used in patients with history of anaphylaxis, urticaria or angioedema to penicillin or ampicillin
	Azithromycin 500 mg

6. Need for post-operative antibiotics after dental procedures

Because of the increased risk of infection, antibiotics may be necessary post-operatively in instances where odontogenic infections need to be addressed.
The regimen of antibiotics prescribed should be discussed with the transplant team.

7. Special concerns about analgesics and narcotics

Different patients would have different specific needs for pain control.
Acetaminophen is to be avoided or used extremely judiciously in view of its potential hepatotoxicity.
Non-steroidal anti-inflammatory drugs are therefore the mainstay of analgesia.
This may lead to increased reliance on opioids for pain control. This should be discussed with the transplant team.
Liver transplant patients have special dental needs. It is important to attend to the oral health aggressively prior to the transplant. The patient should be instructed on oral hygiene and home care both before and after the transplant. These patients would benefit from frequent recalls after the first 6 months of transplant.

28 DENTAL EVALUATION AND MANAGEMENT OF THE PATIENT WITH CHRONIC KIDNEY DISEASE

INTRODUCTION

Chronic kidney disease is defined as the presence of kidney damage or decreased kidney function for 3 or more months. Patients with chronic kidney disease have a higher risk of cardiovascular disease, infection, progression to end-stage renal disease and mortality. The patients have issues with hypertension, volume overload, metabolic disturbances and acid base balance. It is important for the dental professionals to understand the complexity of managing these patients in order to optimize dental management.

1. Medical evaluation of patients with chronic kidney disease

Chronic kidney disease is a heterogeneous group of disorder. In the medical evaluation of the patient presenting with persistent renal disfunction, attempts are made to categorize them by defining the following:

- **Cause of chronic kidney disease**

  Although it is often a constellation of disorders that contribute to the renal dysfunction, being able to define the cause of chronic kidney disease is important in being able to define:
  - Prognosis of disease
  - Projected course of progression
  - Specific treatment options for the disease

- **Staging of chronic kidney disease**

  The glomerular filtration rate (GFR) has been widely used to stage chronic renal disease:
  - G1 GFR >90 mL/min per 1.73 m^2
  - G2 GFR 60 to 89 mL/min per 1.73 m^2
  - G3a GFR 45 to 59 mL/min per 1.73 m^2
  - G3b GFR 30 to 44 mL/min per 1.73 m^2
  - G4 GFR 15 to 29 mL/min per 1.73 m^2
  - G5 GFR less than 15 mL/min per 1.73 m^2 or treatment by dialysis

- **Kidney damage as gauged by degree of albuminuria**

  Renal damage is best gauged by the amount of albumen in the urine, expressed as urinary albumen as a ratio to urinary creatinine (albumen/creatinine ration or ACR)
  - A1 ACR <30 mg/g Normal
  - A2 ACR 30 to 299 mg/g Moderately increased
  - A3 ACR >300 mg/g Severely increased

Knowing the cause of the chronic kidney disease will aid management and planning. The use of GFR and degree of proteinuria will allow accurate depiction of the degree of renal compromise.

2. Medical management of the patient with chronic obstructive pulmonary disease

Patients with chronic kidney disease have a vast array of complications. Defining the cause and degree of renal compromise is important in the selection of therapeutic options.

- **Cause of chronic kidney disease**

  Knowing the cause of the disease can dictate therapeutic options. Some examples:
  - Patients with adult dominant onset polycystic kidney disease are generally treated with tolvaptan, which slows down growth of cysts.
  - Patients with IgA nephropathy may be treated with delayed release capsules of budesonide designed to deliver treatment to an area of the gut thought to play a role in IgA nephropathy.
  - Patients with diabetic nephropathy are treated with angiotensin converting enzyme inhibitor or angiotensin receptor blocker to aggressively control blood pressure.

- **Metabolic complications**

  Patients with chronic kidney disease have a wide array of metabolic disorder necessitating treatment:
  - Hyperkalemia
  - Fluid overload
  - Acid-base disorders
  - Bone mineral disorders

- **Anemia**

  Patients with chronic kidney disease have anemia of chronic disease as a result of decreased erythropoietin production from the kidneys. The patients may be on erythropoietin therapy.

  Patients with chronic kidney disease are also more prone to bleeding complications because of adverse effect of uremia on platelet function. They are therefore also prone to iron-deficiency necessitating iron orally or parenterally.

- **Cardiovascular complications**

  Patients with chronic kidney disease have significant cardiovascular complications necessitating medical intervention:
  - Hypertension necessitating aggressive management to minimize progressive renal decline.
  - Fluid overload with resultant congestive heart failure.
  - Hyperkalemia with resultant issues with arrhythmia.
  - Uremic pericarditis with severe uremia.

- **Bone complications**

  Patients with chronic kidney disease have a wide array of metabolic disorder necessitating treatment:
  - Treatment with vitamin D.
  - Treatment with phosphate binders.

- **Bleeding disorder**

  Patients with chronic kidney disease have abnormal platelet function as a result of uremic environment.

- **Compromised wound healing**

  Patients with chronic kidney disease have compromises to wound healing.

- **Infection**

  Patients with chronic kidney disease have compromised immune response and are therefore more prone to infections.

3. Dental evaluation of the patient with chronic kidney disease

Careful evaluation of the cause of the renal disease, the degree of renal compromise, the medications the patient is on and the current adequacy of control of complications is important for the dental management of the patient with chronic kidney disease.

- **Medical History**

  The patient should be asked about the specifics of the chronic kidney disorder. The degree of renal compromise as reflected by the G stage and the albumen/creatinine ratio will be a good guide as to the severity of the disease and the likelihood of the various attendant complications.

- **Blood and urine tests**

  The most recent CBC and metabolic profile should be reviewed. This will help define the degree of renal dysfunction and the attendant complications.
  The most recent albumen/creatine ratio should be used to assess degree of renal damage.

- **Medications the patient is on**

  All medications the patient is on for chronic kidney disease should be reviewed. This will provide a sense of the many complications the patient may be treated for.

- **Cardiovascular complications**

  History of blood pressure control, history of arrhythmia and history of congestive heart failure should be noted.

- **Bleeding complications**

  The patient should be asked about the specifics of easy bruising and bleeding diathesis. In general, patients with more advanced stages of chronic kidney disease should be assumed to be at higher risk of bleeding complications.

- **Anemia**

  The most recent CBC should be reviewed.
  It should be noted whether the patient is on erythropoietin treatment.

- **History of wound healing**

  Careful attention to blood pressure control, history of arrhythmia and history of congestive heart failure should be paid.

- **History of infection**

  Careful attention to blood pressure control, history of arrhythmia and history of congestive heart failure should be paid.

4. Dental management of the patient with chronic kidney disease

- **Degree of renal dysfunction**

  Elective dentistry should be avoided in all patients with unstable renal function. Particular care should be exercised in the management of patients with stages 4 and 5 renal disease, since they are more prone to hyperkalemia, volume overload, labile hypertension and arrhythmia.

- **Timing of dental procedures**

  The patient should be scheduled for the first appointment of the day, at which time the endogenous catecholamines would be at the highest level.
  The appointments should be short (less than 3 hours) to minimize stress.

- **Medications the patient is on for chronic kidney disease**

  The patient should be instructed to take all of their morning medications on the day of the procedure.

- **Local anesthetic with vasoconstrictors**

  Since the patient is usually already on short-acting or long-acting beta agonist, local anesthetics with vasoconstrictors should be restricted to 2 carpules of 1:100,000 epinephrine or 1:50,000 levonordefrin.

- **Bleeding complications**

  Patients with chronic kidney disease have compromised platelet adhesiveness and are more prone to bleeding complications. Care should be taken to place extra sutures, place compressive packings and dressings, use of microfibrillar collagen hemostat, oxidized thrombin and tranexamic acid. Topical thrombin might be necessary for hemostasis.
  Since patients with chronic kidney disease are generally anemic at baseline, it is important to minimize bleeding so as not to accentuate complications such as congestive heart failure.

- **Post-operative pain control**

  Unfortunately, the mainstays of pain control, non-steroidal anti-inflammatory drugs and COX-2 inhibitors such as celecoxib are absolutely contraindicated.
  Acetaminophen and tramadol may be used for pain control.
  Narcotics should be dosed according to renal function and should be prescribed judiciously.

- **Infection**

  Patients with chronic kidney disease have impaired immune system and are more prone to infection. Antibiotics may be necessary to manage odontogenic infections. Care should be taken to avoid medications that may be nephrotoxic such as minocycline or tetracycline.

- **Wound healing**
  Patients with chronic kidney disease have impaired healing. Care needs to be taken to optimize wound healing.

- **Consultation**
  When in doubt, particularly in patients with stages 3b, 4 and 5 disease, it would be prudent to have medical clearance prior to dental interventions.

Although management of the patient with chronic kidney disease can be quite complicated, the dental professional should lean heavily on the adequacy of control of the many complications for evaluation and management of patient for optimal care. The goal is to exclude patients with unstable renal parameters to elective dental procedure.

29

DENTAL EVALUATION AND MANAGEMENT OF THE PATIENT ON DIALYSIS

INTRODUCTION

Patients with end-stage renal disease require renal replacement therapy. Some patients undergo renal transplantation (Chapter 30), but a significant portion of patients require dialysis, either hemodialysis or peritoneal dialysis. Prevalence of patients on dialysis is increasing in a steady fashion, and it is important for the dental professional to understand their special needs in order to optimize dental therapy in these patients.

1. Medical evaluation of patients on hemodialysis

Ninety percent of patients on dialysis are on hemodialysis. Patients on hemodialysis are generally dialyzed three times a week for 4 hours each session at an outpatient dialysis center. Increasingly, dialysis at home is preferred by patients and physicians and these patients may require dialysis five times a week.

Patients on hemodialysis have vascular accesses to permit access to the circulation. They require systemic anticoagulation with heparin during dialysis to prevent clotting in the dialysis coils. There is usually significant amount of fluid removal during the 4-hour dialysis.

- **Access for dialysis**

  Different accesses can be used for dialysis:

  - Arteriovenous fistula is created by connecting the end of a vein to the side of an artery, either in the radial position or in the brachiocephalic position. This is the most common and the preferred vascular access since it is the least likely access to clot or to get infected. The access takes several months to mature after creation.

- Arteriovenous graft is created by placement of a synthetic graft to connect a vein to an artery. The access is more prone to infection and clotting but can be used shortly after creation.
- Internal jugular catheter: a double lumen catheter can be placed via a subcutaneous tunnel into the internal jugular vein. This is most prone to infection and clotting and is generally only used as a temporary access unless there is no means of establishing an arteriovenous fistula or graft.

- **Anticoagulation during dialysis**

  During hemodialysis, the patient receives systemic heparin so as not to have clots in the dialysis coils or lines. The effect of the anticoagulation persists for hours after dialysis.

- **Volume shifts during dialysis**

  Since the patient is dialyzed intermittently, fluid accumulates in between hemodialysis. During dialysis, 2 to 4 liters of fluid may have to be removed. The volume shift may cause transient hypotension that resolves with time.

2. Medical evaluation of the patient on continuous ambulatory peritoneal dialysis (CAPD) or automated intermittent peritoneal dialysis (AIPD)

A small percentage of patients with chronic kidney disease are on peritoneal dialysis. A catheter is surgically placed in the peritonea cavity. Two to three liters of dialysate are infused into the abdominal cavity, dwell for 4 hours and then drained. Four to six exchanges are done continuously every day, either by the patient (continuous ambulatory peritoneal dialysis, CAPD) or with the use of a cycler overnight (automated intermittent peritoneal dialysis, AIPD). In these modalities, the peritoneal membrane becomes the exchange membrane. The exchanges are conducted by the patient as an outpatient after appropriate training.

The major concerns with peritoneal dialysis are infection, malfunctioning of the catheter and loss of dialysis membrane surface.

- **Concern over infection**

  Despite use of aseptic techniques, infection remains the greatest problem with peritoneal dialysis:

  - Peritonitis can occur and requires aggressive systemic and intraperitoneal antibiotic treatment.
  - Less commonly, the exit site of the catheter can be infected, again requiring systemic antibiotic treatment.

- **Volume shifts during dialysis**

  - Peritoneal dialysis is very effective at volume removal.

- Fluid restriction can often be eliminated in patients on effective peritoneal dialysis.
- Blood pressure medications are often decreased in patients on peritoneal dialysis.

3. Medical management of patients on dialysis

Patients on either hemodialysis or peritoneal dialysis have similar complications necessitating interventions and management:

- **Anemia**

  Patients with chronic kidney disease on dialysis have anemia of chronic disease as a result of decreased erythropoietin production from the kidneys. The patients may be on erythropoietin therapy.

  Patients with chronic kidney disease are also more prone to bleeding complications because of adverse effect of uremia on platelet function. They are therefore also prone to iron-deficiency necessitating iron orally or parenterally.

- **Cardiovascular complications**

  Patients with chronic kidney disease on dialysis have significant cardiovascular complications necessitating medical intervention:
  - Hypertension is generally under better control.
  - Fluid overload with resultant congestive heart failure is also less common.
  - Hyperkalemia with resultant issues with arrhythmia can occur.

- **Bone complications**

  Patients with chronic kidney disease on dialysis have a wide array of metabolic disorder necessitating treatment:
  - Treatment with vitamin D.
  - Treatment of hyperphosphatemia with phosphate binders.

- **Bleeding disorder**

  Patients with chronic kidney disease on dialysis have abnormal platelet function as a result of uremic environment.

- **Compromised wound healing**

  Patients with chronic kidney disease on dialysis have compromises to wound healing.

- **Infection**

  Patients with chronic kidney disease on dialysis have compromised immune response and are therefore more prone to infections.

4. Dental evaluation of the patient on hemodialysis

Specific information should be obtained from the patient on hemodialysis, including the type of access the patient is on, the timing and the duration of dialysis.

- **Medical history**

  The patient should be asked about the specifics of the type of dialysis the patient is on, whether it is done in center or at home.

  The type of access used in dialysis should be noted.

  The timing of the dialysis and the duration of the dialysis should be noted.

  Whether the patient has hemodynamic issues during or after dialysis should be noted.

  In the patient on peritoneal dialysis, the modality of dialysis (CAPD versus AIPD) should be noted.

- **Blood tests**

  The most recent CBC and metabolic profile should be reviewed. This will help define the adequacy of dialysis.

- **Medications the patient is on**

  All medications the patient is on should be reviewed.

- **Cardiovascular complications**

  History of blood pressure control, history of arrhythmia and history of congestive heart failure should be noted.

- **Bleeding complications**

  The patient should be asked about the specifics of easy bruising and bleeding diathesis. In general, patients with more advanced stages of chronic kidney disease should be assumed to be at higher risk of bleeding complications.

- **Anemia**

  The most recent CBC should be reviewed.

  It should be noted whether the patient is on erythropoietin treatment.

- **History of wound healing**

  Careful attention to blood pressure control, history of arrhythmia and history of congestive heart failure should be paid.

- **History of infection**

  Careful attention to blood pressure control, history of arrhythmia and history of congestive heart failure should be paid.

5. Dental evaluation of the patient on peritoneal dialysis

Specific information should be obtained from the patient on peritoneal dialysis:

- **Medical history**

  The patient should be asked about the specifics of the type of peritoneal dialysis the patient is on, whether it is continuous ambulatory peritoneal dialysis or automated intermittent dialysis.

  The timing of the dialysis should be noted.

  Whether the patient has hemodynamic issues during or after dialysis should be noted.

  History and frequency of peritonitis should be noted.

- **Blood tests**

  The most recent CBC and metabolic profile should be reviewed. This will help define the adequacy of dialysis.

- **Medications the patient is on**

  All medications the patient is on should be reviewed.

- **Cardiovascular complications**

  History of blood pressure control, history of arrhythmia and history of congestive heart failure should be noted.

- **Bleeding complications**

  The patient should be asked about the specifics of easy bruising and bleeding diathesis. In general, patients with more advanced stages of chronic kidney disease should be assumed to be at higher risk of bleeding complications.

- **Anemia**

  The most recent CBC should be reviewed.

  It should be noted whether the patient is on erythropoietin treatment.

- **History of wound healing**

  Careful attention to blood pressure control, history of arrhythmia and history of congestive heart failure should be paid.

- **History of infection**

  Careful attention to blood pressure control, history of arrhythmia and history of congestive heart failure should be paid.

6. Dental management of the patient on hemodialysis

- **Timing of dental procedures**

  Since systemic heparin is used during the dialysis procedure, dental procedures should be scheduled on a non-dialysis day.

  The patient should be scheduled for the first appointment of the day, at which time the endogenous catecholamines would be at the highest level.

  The appointments should be short (less than 3 hours) to minimize stress.

- **Medications the patient is on**

  The patient should be instructed to take all of their morning medications on the day of the procedure.

- **Need for antibiotic premedication**

  The need for premedication is predicated upon the dialysis access the patient has

  - Arteriovenous fistula: antibiotic premedication is usually not necessary.
  - Arteriovenous shunt: because of the higher risk of infection, standard antibiotic premedication is usually prescribed.
  - Internal jugular catheter: because of the very high risk of infection, standard antibiotic premedication should be prescribed.

- **Local anesthetic with vasoconstrictors**

  Because of cardiovascular complications in patients on dialysis, local anesthetics with vasoconstrictors should be restricted to 2 carpules of 1:100,000 epinephrine or 1:50,000 levonordefrin.

- **Bleeding complications**

  Patients on hemodialysis have compromised platelet adhesiveness and are more prone to bleeding complications. Care should be taken to place extra sutures, place compressive packings and dressings, use of microfibrillar collagen hemostat, oxidized thrombin and tranexamic acid. Topical thrombin might be necessary for hemostasis.

  Since patients with chronic kidney disease are generally anemic at baseline, it is important to minimize bleeding so as not to accentuate complications such as congestive heart failure.

- **Post-operative pain control**

  Unfortunately, the mainstays of pain control, non-steroidal anti-inflammatory drugs and COX-2 inhibitors such as celecoxib are absolutely contraindicated.

  Acetaminophen and Tramadol may be used for pain control.

  Narcotics should be dosed according to renal function and should be prescribed judiciously.

- **Infection**

  Patients on hemodialysis have impaired immune systems and are more prone to infection. Antibiotics may be necessary to manage odontogenic infections. Care should be taken to avoid medications that may be nephrotoxic, such as minocycline or tetracycline.

- **Wound healing**

  Patients on hemodialysis have impaired healing. Care needs to be taken to optimize wound healing.

- **Consultation**

  When in doubt, it would be prudent to have medical clearance prior to dental interventions.

7. Dental management of the patient on peritoneal dialysis

- **Timing of dental procedures**

  The patient should be scheduled for the first appointment at a time when the endogenous catecholamines would be at the highest level.

  The appointments should be short (less than 3 hours) to minimize stress.

- **Medications the patient is on**

  The patient should be instructed to take all of their morning medications on the day of the procedure.

- **Need for antibiotic premedication**

  Because of concern over transient bacteremia during dentistry causing peritonitis, all patients on peritoneal dialysis should be on antibiotic premedication.

- **Local anesthetic with vasoconstrictors**

  Because of cardiovascular complications in patients on peritoneal dialysis, local anesthetics with vasoconstrictors should be restricted to 2 carpules of 1:100,000 epinephrine or 1:50,000 levonordefrin.

- **Bleeding complications**

  Patients on peritoneal dialysis have compromised platelet adhesiveness and are more prone to bleeding complications. Care should be taken to place extra sutures, place compressive packings and dressings, use of microfibrillar collagen hemostat, oxidized thrombin and tranexamic acid. Topical thrombin might be necessary for hemostasis.

  Since patients on peritoneal dialysis are generally anemic at baseline, it is important to minimize bleeding so as not to accentuate complications such as congestive heart failure.

- **Post-operative pain control**

  Unfortunately, the mainstays of pain control, non-steroidal anti-inflammatory drugs and COX-2 inhibitors such as celecoxib are absolutely contraindicated.
  Acetaminophen and tramadol may be used for pain control.
  Narcotics should be prescribed judiciously in reduced doses.

- **Infection**

  Patients on peritoneal dialysis have impaired immune systems and are more prone to infection. Because of the heightened concerns over peritonitis, antibiotic premedication should be prescribed. Odontogenic infections should be treated aggressively.

- **Wound healing**

  Patients on peritoneal dialysis have impaired healing. Care needs to be taken to optimize wound healing.

- **Consultation**

  When in doubt, it would be prudent to have medical clearance prior to dental interventions.

Although management of the patient on dialysis can be quite complicated, the dental procedures can be carried out through meticulous attention to the specific details of the dialytic process and with consultation with the patient's physician.

30 DENTAL EVALUATION AND MANAGEMENT OF THE PATIENT WITH RENAL TRANSPLANT

INTRODUCTION

Renal transplants are generally regarded as the best modality for management of end stage renal disease in the appropriate patient. Patients can receive their renal transplant from a:

- Living related donor
- Cadaveric donor
- Living unrelated donor

All patients after transplantation will require life-long immunosuppression. They are usually on combinations of drugs working in different paths of immune response:

- Glucocorticoids
- Antimetabolites such as mycophenolate or, less commonly, azathioprine
- Calcineurin inhibitors such as tacrolimus, sirolimus or, less commonly, cyclosporine

Medications the patient is on after renal transplant may have oral complications and may require specific dental attention.

Different transplant programs have different protocols for antibiotic premedication for dental procedures. It is important for the dental professional to get medical clearance from the transplant team to accommodate the special needs of any given patient.

Patients with renal transplants are more prone to infections, including dental infections. It is important to pay heightened attention to the patient's oral health and to use antibiotics for management of odontogenic infections.

1. Dental management of patients before renal transplant

In general, it is recommended that patients not undergo elective dental procedures for the first 6 months after transplant. It is therefore recommended that dental health be optimized as much as possible prior to planned transplant.

- **Dental cleaning**
  It is important to have a thorough dental cleaning before the procedure to optimize oral health going into transplant.

- **Management of gingival disease**
  Gingival hyperplasia is a common complication of some of the immunosuppressive drugs. It is therefore important to treat gingival disease prior to transplant to minimize infection after the transplant.

- **Tooth extractions**
  Any problematic teeth that may cause infection should be extracted prior to transplant.

- **Oral hygiene instructions**
  The patient should be instructed on proper oral hygiene techniques to optimize oral health going into the transplant and after the transplant.

By addressing these oral health issues before the renal transplant, the patient should have fewer complications after the transplant when dental interventions would be significantly more complicated.

2. Dental management for the first 6 months after transplant

Except for extenuating circumstances, it is important to avoid elective dental procedures for the first 6 months after transplant. Immunosuppressive drugs tend to be at the highest level during this period, thereby interfering with wound healing and increasing the likelihood of infection.

In instances where dental procedures have to be done, it is important to consult the transplant team in order to assess the need for antibiotic premedication and post-operative antibiotics. It is important to discuss medications that may need to be prescribed peri-operatively in order to minimize the likelihood of drug-drug interactions.

3. Dental management of the patient after 6 months post-transplant

It is important to aggressively address oral health of the patient following renal transplant. The patients are more prone to oral infections, which can result in systemic infection that can greatly complicate the patient's welfare.

- **Oral hygiene instructions**
  The patient should be instructed on proper oral hygiene techniques to optimize oral health.

- **Dental cleaning**
  Frequent recalls are appropriate in these patients in order to optimize oral health.

- **Management of gingival disease**
  Gingival hyperplasia is a common complication of some of the immunosuppressive drugs, particularly cyclosporine.
  Meticulous home oral health care and frequent recalls will minimize this complication.

4. Dental implications of immunosuppressive drugs

Medications commonly prescribed after transplant can have important dental implications. In general, infections are more common on immunosuppressive drugs. It is also important to understand that medications the dental professional may prescribe can have drug-drug interactions with the immunosuppressive drugs and can interfere with their efficacy.
It is important to connect with the transplant team prior to elective interventions to coordinate the optimal management of the patient.

- **Steroids**
  Steroids are commonly prescribed after a transplant. The dose of steroids is weaned rapidly during the first months after transplant. Adrenal insufficiency is generally not an issue beyond the first 6 months after transplant and stress dose steroids are generally not necessary.
  However, steroids do impair healing and increase the likelihood of infection.
  It is important that you address these issues with the transplant team to be sure that there is no need for adjustment of the steroid dose.

- **Tacrolimus**
  Tacrolimus can cause mild gingival hyperplasia. It can also cause xerostomia. Both conditions can promote gingival inflammation, infection and tooth decay.

- **Sirolimus**
  Sirolimus can lead to oral ulcers, which need to be addressed with topical management.
  Sirolimus can also cause xerostomia, which can lead to infection and tooth decay.

- **Mycophenolate**
  Mycophenolate can cause xerostomia.

- **Cyclosporine**
  Cyclosporine can cause significant gingival hyperplasia. Fortunately, cyclosporine has been progressively phased out, yielding to the newer immunosuppressants.

5. Need for antibiotic premedication for dental procedures

There are no specific guidelines that are uniformly adopted. Different transplant centers have different protocols. It is therefore important to discuss the need for premedication with the transplant team prior to elective surgery.

If antibiotic premedication is deemed necessary, amoxicillin 2 g should be given an hour before the planned procedure to patients without penicillin allergy **(Table 30.1)**.

For patients with penicillin allergy, cephalexin 2 g should be given an hour before the planned procedure. Cephalexin should not be used in patients with a history of anaphylaxis, urticaria or angioedema to penicillin or ampicillin **(Table 30.1)**.

TABLE 30.1 Antibiotics for premedication in renal transplant patients

Premedication given one hour before procedure	
No penicillin allergy	**Penicillin allergy**
Amoxicillin 2 g	Cephalexin 2 g Should not be used in patients with history of anaphylaxis, urticaria or angioedema to penicillin or ampicillin
	Azithromycin 500 mg

6. Need for post-operative antibiotics after dental procedures

Because of the increased risk of infection, antibiotics may be necessary post-operatively in instances where odontogenic infections need to be addressed.

The regimen of antibiotics prescribed should be discussed with the transplant team.

7. Special concerns about analgesics and narcotics

Different patients would have different specific needs for pain control.

In general, acetaminophen remains the foundation of analgesia in patients with renal transplant, whereas non-steroidal anti-inflammatory drugs are to be avoided in patients after renal transplant.

This may lead to increased reliance on opioids for pain control. This should be discussed with the transplant team.

Renal transplant patients have special dental needs. It is important to attend to the oral health aggressively prior to the transplant. The patient should be instructed on oral hygiene and home care both before and after the transplant. These patients would benefit from frequent recalls after the first 6 months of transplant.

31 DENTAL EVALUATION AND MANAGEMENT OF THE PATIENT ON ANTICOAGULANTS

INTRODUCTION

An increasing number of patients are on oral anticoagulants. The most common reason is for the management of the patient with chronic or intermittent atrial fibrillation. Adequate anticoagulation is critical to prevent embolic strokes in this population. Similarly, patients with prosthetic valves may require anticoagulation, either transiently or indefinitely.
Other indications for anticoagulation may be to prevent the recurrence of deep venous thrombophlebitis or pulmonary embolization. Short-term anticoagulation may be prescribed after certain orthopedic procedures such as hip and knee surgeries. In some instances, anticoagulation may be necessary because of an inherent risk of clotting and hypercoagulable states, such as anti-phospholipid antibody syndrome.

There are two major categories of anticoagulants:

- Coumadin (warfarin), which interferes with vitamin K dependent coagulation factors.
- Direct oral anticoagulants (DOACs), which interferes with the last part of the coagulation pathway, either thrombin or factor X.

It is important to understand the indication for anticoagulation in each patient, the anticoagulant used in order to assess the risk of bleeding from the dental procedure done and the risk of clotting and embolic events if the anticoagulation is interrupted.

1. Dental evaluation of the patient on Coumadin

Use of Coumadin is decreasing in view of the increasing use of direct oral anticoagulants (DOACs), but it continues to be important in certain patients.

Patients on Coumadin have frequent testing of prothrombin time/international normalized ratio (PT/INR) to measure adequacy of anticoagulation. PT/INR is generally maintained at a therapeutic level of between 2 and 3. In some circumstances where a high degree of anticoagulation is desired, the patient may need higher PT/INR (2.5 to 3.5)

- **Atrial fibrillation, deep venous thrombophlebitis, pulmonary embolism**
    - Increasingly, the use of Coumadin has been supplanted by the use of the direct oral anticoagulants (DOACs) for these indications.
    - DOACs are equal to Coumadin in efficacy.
    - There are fewer bleeding complications from DOACs.
    - In these patients, PT/INR is generally maintained at a therapeutic range between 2 and 3.

- **Mechanical cardiac valves**
    - These valves are highly thrombogenic.
    - Coumadin therapy is maintained indefinitely.
    - PT/INR is generally maintained at 2.5 to 3.5.
    - Risk of interruption of anticoagulation is high.
    - In general, there is a trend to use biosynthetic valves as opposed to mechanical valves.

- **Biosynthetic heart valves**
    - Valves are made from a combination of biological and synthetic materials. The biological component is usually derived from animal tissues, such as porcine or bovine tissues. The synthetic component of biosynthetic valves is often made from materials such as polyester or polytetrafluoroethylene (PTFE).
    - Patients may be on anticoagulation for a period of time or may require lifelong anticoagulation.

- **Hypercoagulable state: factor V Leiden mutation**
    - Patients can have a genetic mutation in factor V.
    - It is an autosomal dominant disorder.
    - This mutation increases the risk of venous thrombosis.
    - The predisposition to clot formation is variable from patient to patient, but precipitating factors may include pregnancy, oral contraceptive use, hormone replacement therapy and prolonged periods of immobility.
    - Because the tendency of clotting is only slightly increased, many patients with factor V Leiden mutation may be taking anticoagulation under specific circumstances such as long-distance travel.

- **Hypercoagulable state: anti-phospholipid antibody syndrome (APLS)**
    - An autoimmune disorder with antibodies targeting proteins in the coagulation cascade, creating increased risks of clotting.
    - It can be a primary condition or in association with other autoimmune diseases such as systemic lupus erythematosus.
    - Patients can have recurrent blood clots with predisposition to deep venous thrombophlebitis, pulmonary emboli or embolic strokes.
    - Patients can also have complications during pregnancy, such as miscarriage, preeclampsia or impaired fetal growth.
    - Patients are often treated with Coumadin.
    - PT/INR may be maintained at the higher therapeutic range of 2.5 to 3.5.
    - Interruption of anticoagulation may be problematic.

2. Dental management of the patient on Coumadin

In all patients on Coumadin, PT/INR should be determined within 2-3 days of the planned procedure so as to be able to ascertain the risk of bleeding.

It is important to balance the risk of bleeding against the risk of clot formation.

Interruption of Coumadin is not a minor undertaking, since it takes 3-4 days for the PT/INR to come down and it takes 3-4 days for the PT/INR to return to therapeutic range after resumption of anticoagulation. Randomized trials have indicated that the risk of embolic stroke outweighs the benefit of transient interruption of Coumadin therapy.

In general, routine dental procedures such as dental hygiene, fillings or simple extractions can usually be performed without interruption of Coumadin therapy, provided that the PT/INR is in the therapeutic range of 2-3.

In procedures where hemostasis is a concern, interruption of Coumadin therapy should be done in consultation with the patient's physician since **short-term bridging** might be necessary. In this instance, Coumadin is stopped and the patient is placed on low-molecular weight heparin by injection twice a day. This is continued until the PT/INR is back in therapeutic range after resumption of Coumadin.

- **Atrial fibrillation, deep venous thrombophlebitis, pulmonary embolism**
    - In general, interruption of Coumadin therapy is not warranted.
    - However, in instances where there are concerns about hemostasis, minor adjustments of the Coumadin dosing might be helpful: if the PT/INR is greater than 2.5, holding a single dose of Coumadin the night before the dental intervention might be appropriate since it will get the INR closer to 2, but the patient would still be in therapeutic range. This should be done in consultation with the patient's physician.
    - If there is great concern about bleeding complications, the patient may need bridging therapy, in consultation with the patient's physician.

- **Mechanical cardiac valves**
  - Because of the high risk of clotting complications, the patient should be kept on anticoagulation.
  - This should not pose a significant problem for routine dentistry such as dental hygiene, endodontic procedures or simple extraction.
  - In instances where significant bleeding is anticipated, the patient will need bridging therapy in consultation with the patient's physician.

- **Biosynthetic heart valves**
  - These patients may be on anticoagulation for the first 6 months after placement of the valves.
  - During the first 6 months, anticoagulation should not be interrupted.
    - This should not pose a significant problem for routine dentistry such as dental hygiene, endodontic procedures or simple extraction.
    - In instances where significant bleeding is anticipated, the patient will need bridging therapy, in consultation with the patient's physician.
  - Beyond the first 6 months after valve placement, anticoagulation is often not necessary.

- **Hypercoagulable state: factor V Leiden mutation**
  - These patients are often not on chronic anticoagulation.
  - If they are on Coumadin and are in therapeutic range (INR 2-3), the majority of the dental procedures can be done without interruption of Coumadin.
  - In instances where significant bleeding is anticipated, the patient will need bridging therapy, in consultation with the patient's physician.

- **Hypercoagulable state: anti-phospholipid antibody syndrome (APLS)**
  - Not infrequently, PT/INR may be maintained at the higher therapeutic range of 2.5 to 3.5.
  - Because of the high risk of clotting complications, interruption of anticoagulation should be done only with consultation with the patient's physician since bridging therapy will be necessary.

3. Drug-Drug interaction for patients on Coumadin

- **Antibiotics**
  - Coumadin interferes with vitamin K dependent coagulation factors.
  - Vitamin K is synthesized by bacteria in the colon and antibiotics can decrease the systemic vitamin K level and cause prolongation of PT/INR.
  - Whenever antibiotics are prescribed for odontogenic infections, it is important to check a repeat PT/INR in 3-4 days after the initiation of antibiotics to make sure that there is no prolongation of PT/INR. The patient's physician should be alerted to make changes in the Coumadin dosing if there is PT/INR prolongation.

- **Non-steroidal anti-inflammatory drugs**
    - Should be avoided in patients on Coumadin in order not to cause bleeding complications, particularly gastrointestinal bleeding.
    - Alternatives such as tramadol and opioid may be necessary for pain control.

- **Steroids**
  Should be avoided in patients on Coumadin in order not to cause bleeding complications, particularly gastrointestinal bleeding.

4. Direct oral anticoagulants (DOACs)

Increasingly, the direct oral anticoagulants have replaced Coumadin as the major anticoagulant of choice. With some exceptions, such as in patients with mechanical cardiac valves or antiphospholipid antibody syndrome, the DOACs are actually the first line therapy as anticoagulants.
All of the DOACs are designed to inhibit the coagulation pathway late in the formation of a clot, either as a thrombin inhibitor or as an inhibitor of factor Xa function.

There are four DOACs in clinical use:

- **Dabigatrin (Pradaxa)**
    - Direct thrombin inhibitor.
    - Given twice a day.
    - Renally excreted.
    - Idarucizumab (Praxbind), a monoclonal antibody against dabigatran, is a specific antidote for the reversal of bleeding in a patient on dabigatran.

- **Rivaroxaban (Xarelto)**
    - Inhibitor of factor Xa.
    - Given once a day, usually at night.
    - Renally excreted.
    - Andexanet alfa (Andexxa), a decoy factor X Fc protein, is a specific antidote for the reversal of bleeding in a patient on rivaroxaban.

- **Apixaban (Eliquis)**
    - Inhibitor of factor Xa.
    - Given twice a day.
    - NOT renally excreted.
    - Preferred DOACs in patients with renal compromise.
    - Andexanet alfa (Andexxa), a decoy factor X Fc protein, is a specific antidote for the reversal of bleeding in a patient on apixaban.

- **Edoxaban (Savaysa, Lixana, Roteas)**
  - Inhibitor of factor Xa.
  - Given once a day, usually at night.
  - Renally excreted.
  - Andexanet alfa (Andexxa), a decoy factor X Fc protein, is a specific antidote for the reversal of bleeding in a patient on apixaban.

5. Dental evaluation of the patient on direct oral anticoagulants (DOACs)

- **Atrial fibrillation, deep venous thrombophlebitis, pulmonary embolism**
  - Increasingly, the use of Coumadin has been supplanted by the use of the new direct oral anticoagulants (DOACs) for these indications.
  - DOACs are equal to Coumadin in its efficacy.
  - There are fewer bleeding complications from DOACs.

- **Mechanical cardiac valves**
  - These valves are highly thrombogenic.
  - Coumadin therapy is still the mainstay of anticoagulation in these patients.

- **Biosynthetic heart valves**
  - These valves are thrombogenic in the first 6 months.
  - Patients are generally on Coumadin instead of DOAC during the 6 months.
  - Patients may be off of anticoagulation altogether beyond the first 6 months as the valve is endothelialized.

- **Hypercoagulable state: factor V Leiden mutation**
  - Patients may not be on anticoagulants at all.
  - DOAC is increasingly the drug of choice for short-term anticoagulation (e.g., for long distance travel).

- **Hypercoagulable state: anti-phospholipid antibody syndrome (APLS)**
  - Patients are generally treated with Coumadin.
  - PT/INR may be maintained at the higher therapeutic range of 2.5 to 3.5.
  - Interruption of anticoagulation may be problematic.

6. Dental management of the patient on direct oral anticoagulants (DOACs)

It is important to balance the risk of bleeding against the risk of clot formation.

In general, routine dental procedures such as dental hygiene, fillings or simple extractions can usually be performed without interruption of DOAC therapy.

In procedures where hemostasis is a concern, minor adjustments of DOAC therapy should be done in consultation with the patient's physician.
In instances where excessive bleeding is a concern, interruption of DOAC therapy should be done in consultation with the patient's physician and decision about short-term bridging therapy may be necessary in rare cases.

- **Atrial fibrillation, deep venous thrombophlebitis, pulmonary embolism**
  - In general, interruption of DOAC therapy is not warranted.
  - However, in instances where there are concerns about hemostasis, minor adjustments of the new DOAC dosing might be helpful:
    - ❑ For dabigatran and apixaban, the dose the night before the procedure and the dose on the morning of the procedure can be held with resumption of therapy the evening after the procedure.
    - ❑ For rivaroxaban and edoxaban, the dose the night before the procedure can be held with resumption of therapy the evening after the procedure.
  - If there is great concern about bleeding complications, the patient may need bridging therapy in consultation with the patient's physician.

- **Mechanical cardiac valves**
  - These patients are generally on Coumadin.

- **Biosynthetic heart valves**
  - These patients may be on DOAC for the first 6 months after placement of the valves.
  - During the first 6 months, anticoagulation should not be interrupted.
    - ❑ This should not pose a significant problem for routine dentistry such as dental hygiene, endodontic procedures or simple extraction.
    - ❑ In instances where significant bleeding is anticipated, the patient will need bridging therapy, in consultation with the patient's physician.
  - Beyond the first 6 months after valve placement, anticoagulation is often not necessary.

- **Hypercoagulable state: factor V Leiden mutation**
  - These patients are often not on chronic anticoagulation.
  - If they are on DOAC, anticoagulation can be interrupted with consultation with the patient's physician since they are at low risk of forming clots.

- **Hypercoagulable state: anti-phospholipid antibody syndrome (APLS)**
  - These patients are generally on Coumadin.

For the dental professional, care should be directed at the reason for anticoagulation, the specific type of anticoagulation used, the risk of clotting in any given patient and the risk of bleeding from any specific dental intervention. Careful coordination with the patient's physician is important for successful management of these patients.

32 DENTAL EVALUATION AND MANAGEMENT OF THE PATIENT ON ANTI-PLATELET THERAPY

INTRODUCTION

An increasing number of patients are on anti-platelet therapy. In general, anti-platelet therapy is designed to prevent clotting in the arterial side of the circulation, whereas anticoagulants such as Coumadin and direct oral anticoagulants (DOACs) are used for clotting in a lower flow system such as the venous system and the left atrial appendage. Anticoagulation therapy should be used in patients with atrial fibrillation, deep venous thrombophlebitis, pulmonary embolism or hypercoagulable states or as prophylaxis against deep venous thrombophlebitis and pulmonary embolism in the post-operative period.

Anti-platelet therapy should be used in patients after a myocardial infarction or stroke to prevent recurrence and in patients with a variety of stents in place, particularly coronary artery stents.

In patients with cardiac stents, double anti-platelet therapy may be in place for the first 6 to 12 months, and bleeding complications can indeed occur. The dental professional needs to weigh the risk of bleeding against the risk of clotting in every clinical situation and should consult the patient's physician before alteration in anti-platelet therapy is contemplated.

Three anti-platelet agents are used clinically:

- **Aspirin** is generally the mainstay of all anti-platelet therapy in doses of 81 mg to 325 mg each day.
- **Clopidogrel (Plavix)** is often the agent of choice for patients in need of double anti-platelet therapy after coronary interventions.

- **Ticagrelor (Brilinta)** is increasingly chosen after coronary intervention because of improved cardiac outcome in patients with acute coronary syndrome in comparison to clopidogrel.

1. Dental evaluation of the patient on anti-platelet therapy

The indication for the use of anti-platelet therapy is important in the decisions about alteration of anti-platelet therapy for dental intervention. In general, changes are not indicated for routine dentistry such as oral hygiene, endodontic procedures and extractions. However, changes may be indicated in instances where significant bleeding is anticipated, particularly if the patient is on double anti-platelet therapy.
Clinical circumstances where anti-platelet therapy is generally deployed include:

- **Coronary stents: bare metal stents**
  - Percutaneous coronary intervention is very common, and most of the interventions include angioplasty and placement of a stent.
  - After the deployment of a stent, double anti-platelet therapy is usually prescribed for a short period before converting to single anti-platelet therapy using aspirin alone.
  - Bare metal stents have the advantage of a shorter duration of the need for double-anti-platelet therapy (less than 6 months).
  - Bare metal stents have the disadvantage of having restenosis of the stented area because of progressive endothelialization.
  - Bare metal stents are used in patients who are at risk of bleeding complications.

- **Coronary stent: drug-eluting stent**
  - More commonly, a drug-eluting stent is placed after percutaneous coronary intervention.
  - These stents have an antiproliferative agent impregnated into the scaffolding of the stent: sirolimus or paclitaxel. These drugs inhibit the growth of cells in the stent that can cause restenosis.
  - However, the drug-eluting stents carry a higher risk of stent thrombosis (clotting) in comparison to the bare metal stents, particularly in the setting of discontinuation of double anti-platelet therapy.
  - Anti-platelet therapy is generally continued for at least 6 months after the placement of a drug-eluting stent and can be prescribed for a much longer period of time, particularly when multiple stents have been placed.
  - Because of the concern over stent thrombosis, physicians may be more reluctant to discontinue double anti-platelet therapy in these patients.

- **Peripheral vascular stent**
  - Anti-platelet therapy is often prescribed in patients with stents in the peripheral vasculature.

- The stents can be bare metal or drug-eluting stents.
- Double anti-platelet therapy is usually prescribed for the first 6 months after stent placement.
- Conversion to single anti-platelet therapy at 6 months with continuation of aspirin indefinitely unless there is a specific contraindication.

- **Endovascular grafts**
  - Endovascular grafts are placed to improve circulation in patients with vascular stenoses.
  - These grafts can be placed percutaneously in the aorta to bypass aortic stenosis.
  - Anti-platelet therapy is often prescribed in patients with endovascular grafts.
  - Double anti-platelet therapy is usually prescribed for the first 6 months after stent placement.
  - Conversion to single anti-platelet therapy at 6 months with continuation of aspirin indefinitely unless there is a specific contraindication.

- **After myocardial infarction**
  - Anti-platelet therapy with aspirin is uniformly prescribed in patients after a myocardial infarction.
  - Use of anti-platelet therapy significantly decreases the risk of another myocardial infarction.
  - Anti-platelet therapy with aspirin is continued indefinitely unless there is a contraindication.

- **After strokes**
  - In patients with a documented embolic stroke, anticoagulation is generally prescribed.
  - Anti-platelet therapy with aspirin is prescribed in patients with all other forms of stroke.
  - Use of anti-platelet therapy significantly decreases the risk of another stroke.
  - Anti-platelet therapy with aspirin is continued indefinitely unless there is a contraindication.

2. Dental management of the patient on anti-platelet therapy

It is important to balance the risk of bleeding against the risk of clot formation.
In general, routine dental procedures such as dental hygiene, fillings or simple extractions can be performed without interruption of anti-platelet therapy.
In general, single anti-platelet therapy with aspirin pose minimal risk of bleeding.
However, double anti-platelet therapy with aspirin plus clopidogrel/ticagrelor is associated with significant bleeding risk. Whenever it is clinically feasible, a brief period of conversion to single anti-platelet therapy will greatly facilitate hemostasis. This has to

be done in consultation with the patient's physician since they are in a much better position to assess the risk of the conversion.

- **Coronary stents: bare metal stents**
  - Since coronary stents are generally placed in the setting of acute coronary syndrome or an evolving myocardial infarction, elective dental surgery should be deferred for the first 6 months.
  - Beyond 6 months, the patient is generally on single anti-platelet therapy.
  - Dental procedures can proceed with special attention to hemostasis in patients on single anti-platelet therapy.

- **Coronary stent: drug-eluting stent**
  - Since coronary stents are generally placed in the setting of acute coronary syndrome or an evolving myocardial infarction, elective dental surgery should be deferred for the first 6 months.
  - Because of concern over late stent thrombosis, many patients may be on double anti-platelet therapy beyond the first 6 months.
  - Routine dentistry such as dental hygiene, endodontic procedures and simple extraction can proceed under double anti-platelet therapy.
  - In instances where significant bleeding is anticipated, the dental professional should consult with the patient's cardiologist to see if the patient can be on transient single anti-platelet coverage:
    - ❑ Discontinue aspirin while maintaining clopidogrel/ticagrelor for 7 days prior to the dental procedure.
    - ❑ Resume double anti-platelet therapy on the day after the procedure.
  - Careful attention to hemostasis.

- **Peripheral vascular stent**
  - Patients are generally on double anti-platelet therapy for the first 6 months. Elective dental interventions should be deferred until the patient is converted to single anti-platelet therapy.
  - Routine dentistry such as dental hygiene, endodontic procedures and simple extraction can proceed under double anti-platelet therapy.
  - In instances where significant bleeding is anticipated in a patient needing dental intervention despite being on double anti-platelet therapy, the dental professional should consult with the patient's cardiologist to see if the patient can be on transient single anti-platelet coverage:
    - ❑ Discontinue aspirin while maintaining clopidogrel/ticagrelor for 7 days prior to the dental procedure.
    - ❑ Resume double anti-platelet therapy on the day after the procedure.
  - Careful attention to hemostasis.

- **Endovascular grafts**
    - Double anti-platelet therapy is usually prescribed for the first 6 months after stent placement and elective dental intervention should be deferred until the patient is on single anti-platelet therapy.
    - Routine dentistry such as dental hygiene, endodontic procedures and simple extraction can proceed under double anti-platelet therapy.
    - In instances where significant bleeding is anticipated in a patient needing dental intervention despite being on double anti-platelet therapy, the dental professional should consult with the patient's cardiologist to see if the patient can be on transient single anti-platelet coverage:
        - Discontinue aspirin while maintaining clopidogrel/ticagrelor for 7 days prior to the dental procedure.
        - Resume double anti-platelet therapy on the day after the procedure.
    - Careful attention to hemostasis.

- **After myocardial infarction**
    - It is still conventional teaching that elective dental procedures, except for dental hygiene, should be deferred until 6 months after a myocardial infarction in order to minimize cardiovascular risks.
    - Since the patient is on single anti-platelet therapy beyond the first 6 months, dentistry can proceed using normal protocol.

- **After strokes**

  Since the patient is on single anti-platelet therapy beyond the first 6 months, dentistry can proceed using normal protocol.

For the dental professional, care should be directed at the reason for anti-platelet therapy, the specific modality of anti-platelet therapy used, the risk of clotting in any given patient and the risk of bleeding from any specific dental intervention. Careful coordination with the patient's physician is important for successful management of these patients.

33

DENTAL EVALUATION AND MANAGEMENT OF PATIENTS ON IMMUNOTHERAPY

INTRODUCTION

Increasingly, immunotherapy has transformed and become an integral part of management of the patient with cancer. Although there are numerous ways of interfering with the immune response in cancer therapy, treatment with immune checkpoint inhibitors is the most common form of immunotherapy.

Immune-related adverse events are common and can involve virtually every organ. Dental professionals should be attuned to the management of oral complications from immunotherapy.

1. Oral complications of immunotherapy

A number of oral complications have been causally linked with immunotherapy. Pre-existing poor oral health, periodontal disease and caries considerably increase these complications.

- **Mucositis**
  - Mucositis can occur with immunotherapy, but its prevalence is lower than observed with chemotherapy.
  - Mucositis can be graded according to its severity **(Table 33.1)**.

TABLE 33.1 Grading of severity of mucositis

0	No oral mucositis
1	Erythema and soreness
2	Ulcers, able to eat solid food
3	Ulcers, but requires liquid diet
4	Ulcers, unable to tolerate solid or liquid diet

- **Lichen planus**
  - A common oral complication of immunotherapy.
  - A range of clinical manifestations affecting buccal mucosa, tongue and gingiva:
    - White reticularis
    - Erythema
    - Ulcers
  - Severity of lichen planus can similarly be graded.

- **Bullous lesions: bullous pemphigus and mucous membrane pemphigoid**
  - A small percentage of patients on check point inhibitors may develop blistering complications:
    - Bullous pemphigus in the majority of the cases.
    - Less commonly, mucous membrane pemphigoid.
  - Lesions may involve the buccal mucosa, soft palate and tongue.
  - Desquamative gingivitis can be seen in some cases.

- **Erythema multiforme**
  - Infrequent oral complication.
  - Often with concurrent cutaneous manifestation.
  - Multiple intra-oral ulcers and erosions.
  - Hemorrhagic crusting of the lips.

- **Stevens-Johnson syndrome and toxic epidermal necrolysis**
  - The most dreaded mucocutaneous complication.
  - Prodromal skin rashes, followed by mucosal and skin denudation.
  - Painful ulcerations and erosions.
  - Hemorrhagic crusting of the lips.

- **Infectious complications**
  - Altered mucosal membrane as a result of chemotherapy can result in entry of pathogens into the bloodstream, causing systemic complications.

- Altered immune response due to chemotherapy can increase the risk of periodontitis, caries and dental abscesses.

- **Salivary gland dysfunction**
  - Xerostomia can be a complication of immunotherapy.
  - Xerostomia can result in development of caries.
  - Xerostomia can promote oral infection.

2. Prophylactic oral care in patients about to undertake immunotherapy

If feasible, a comprehensive oral examination should be carried out before initiation of immunotherapy.

Aggressive preventive oral care has been important in preventing oral complications when immunotherapy is initiated.

Scaling and root planning, treatment of caries and endodontic therapy should be undertaken. Aggressive management of pulpal, periapical disease and periodontal disease should be done when feasible.

Unsalvageable teeth should be extracted.

It is also understood that prophylactic oral care may not be feasible because of time constraints. Nonetheless, as much preventive oral care as can be done should be undertaken.

3. Management of oral complications of immunotherapy

- **Mucositis**
  - Usually self-limited and does not require treatment.
  - Treatment, when indicated can consist of:
    - "Miracle Mouthwash": topical anesthetics (lidocaine) may be combined with an antacid suspension with or without nystatin in a cocktail.
    - Doxepin rinse.
    - Benzydamine rinse: a nonsteroidal anti-inflammatory agent given as an oral rinse.
    - Mucoadhesive hydrogel can be used as a palliative barrier over injured mucosa.
    - Palifermin may accelerate epithelial restoration.
  - Prevention of mucositis can be helpful with use of:
    - Cryotherapy.
    - Palifermin.
    - Low level laser therapy (Photobiomodulation).

- **Lichen planus**
  - Responds well to topical steroids.
  - Severe cases may require systemic steroids.

- In some instances of severe involvement, immunotherapy may need to be interrupted.

- **Bullous lesions: bullous pemphigus and mucous membrane pemphigoid**
  - Responds to topical steroids.
  - Severe cases may require systemic steroids.
  - Immunosuppressants such as azathioprine, mycophenolate and methotrexate may be used to spare systemic steroid use.
  - In some instances of sever involvement, immunotherapy may need to be interrupted.

- **Erythema multiforme**
  - Topical steroids as first intervention.
  - Systemic steroids if necessary.
  - Empiric antiviral therapy.

- **Stevens-Johnson syndrome and toxic epidermal necrolysis**
  - Associated with significant morbidity and mortality.
  - Usually requires hospitalization.
  - Often managed in ICU or burn units.
  - Systemic steroids.
  - Systemic immunosuppressants.
  - Cessation of immunotherapy.

- **Oral infection**
  - Pockets of infection should be drained and eliminated.
  - Periodontitis should be aggressively addressed.
  - Caries should be aggressively managed.
  - Abscesses should be drained and treated.
  - Judicious use of antibiotics when deemed necessary.

- **Salivary gland dysfunction**
  - Maintain good hydration.
  - Oral hygiene and dental self-care.
  - Monitor for occurrence of oral candidiasis.
  - Use of muscarinic agonist:
    - Pilocarpine
    - Cevimeline

Immunotherapy is increasingly a critical part of cancer management. It is associated with a myriad of oral complications that the dental professionals need to recognize and manage.

34 DENTAL EVALUATION AND MANAGEMENT OF THE PATIENT AFTER HEAD AND NECK RADIATION

INTRODUCTION

Head and neck cancer can be treated with surgery, radiation and head and neck radiation. However, head and neck irradiation is often an important adjunct of treatment. Patients with head and neck radiation present with special oral complications. Dental professionals should be attuned to the prevention and management of these oral complications.

1. Oral complications of head and neck radiation

A number of oral complications have been causally linked with head and neck radiation. Pre-existing poor oral health, periodontal disease and caries considerably increase these complications. Aggressive oral care is important for successful management of these complications.

- **Mucositis**
  - **Mucositis** is the most common complication secondary to head and neck radiation and can be quite debilitating.
  - Generalized erythema begins soon after initiation of radiation therapy.
  - Progressive mucosal breakdown results in desquamation and ulceration.
  - The buccal, labial and lingual mucosae are most commonly affected.
  - The mucosa can be very painful, making eating difficult.
  - Movement of the jaw is also compromised because of pain.
  - Healing of these lesions occurs rapidly after cessation of radiation.
  - Mucositis can be graded to reflect severity of involvement **(Table 34.1).**

TABLE 34.1 Grading of severity of mucositis

Grade	Description
0	No oral mucositis
1	Erythema and soreness
2	Ulcers, able to eat solid food
3	Ulcers, but requires liquid diet
4	Ulcers, unable to tolerate solid or liquid diet

- **Salivary gland dysfunction**
  - Shortly after initiation of radiation, fibroblast proliferation in the salivary glands is noted, leading to eventual, progressive degeneration of the acinar epithelium.
  - Xerostomia is a common complication of head and neck radiation.
  - Xerostomia develops at doses of 1000 to 1500 cGy and occurs toward the end of the first week of therapy.
  - Xerostomia can affect the ability of the patient to eat.
  - Normal saliva serves several bacteriostatic functions, xerostomia results in increased formation of plaques.
  - Xerostomia can result in bacterial colonization and development of caries.
  - Xerostomia can promote oral infection.

- **Infectious complications**
  - Altered mucosal membrane due to head and neck radiation can result in entry of pathogens into the bloodstream, causing systemic complications.
  - Altered immune response due to head and neck radiation can increase the risk of periodontitis, caries and dental abscesses.

- **Oral candidiasis**
  - Candida is a common superinfection in patients with mucositis.
  - Aggressive treatment is necessary to prevent seeding of the bloodstream from this source.

- **Reactivation of herpes simplex virus**

  Patients with pre-existing oral herpes simplex virus are prone to reactivation during head and neck radiation.

- **Radiation caries**
  - Rampant caries occur in patients receiving head and neck radiation.
  - Xerostomia, accelerated decalcification of the irradiated teeth and suboptimal oral hygiene all play a role.
  - Induce subsequent pulpal degeneration and infection.

- **Osteoradionecrosis**
  - Serious complication as a result of fibrotic thickening of blood vessels, replacement of the marrow with connective tissue and subsequent inability to form new bone.
  - 90% occur in the mandible.
  - Recognize the patients most at risk:
    - Radiation dose greater than 5000 cGy.
    - Dentulous patients with poor oral hygiene.
    - Implants for radiation carries a greater risk of osteoradionecrosis than external beam radiation.
    - Ill-fitting prosthesis.
    - Dentulous patients with pre-existing dental disease.
  - Use of high-energy sources of radiation reduces the likelihood of this complication.

2. Prophylactic oral care in patients on head and neck radiation

If feasible, a comprehensive oral examination should be carried out before initiation of head and neck radiation.

Aggressive preventive oral care has been important in preventing oral complications when head and neck radiation is initiated.

Scaling and root planning, treatment of caries and endodontic therapy should be undertaken. Aggressive management of pulpal, periapical disease and periodontal disease should be done when feasible.

Unsalvageable teeth should be extracted.

It is also understood that prophylactic oral care may not be feasible because of time constraints. Nonetheless, as much preventive oral care as can be done should be undertaken.

3. Management of oral complications of head and neck radiation

- **Mucositis**
  - The objectives are palliation and reduction of secondary infection.
  - Palliation of symptoms:
    - "Miracle mouthwash": topical anesthetics (lidocaine) may be combined with an antacid suspension with or without nystatin in a cocktail.
    - Lidocaine in the form of viscous lidocaine as a rinse.
    - Benzocaine in Orabase as a rinse.
    - Dyclonine hydrochloride (Dyclone) as a rinse.
    - Doxepin rinse.
    - Benzydamine rinse: a nonsteroidal anti-inflammatory agent given as an oral rinse.
    - Mucoadhesive hydrogel can be used as a palliative barrier over injured mucosa.
    - Palifermin may accelerate epithelial restoration.

- Candidiasis is the most common secondary infection.
    - Nystatin suspension (400,000 to 600,000 units) four times a day; swish and swallow.
    - Use of clotrimazole troches 10 mg up to five times a day.
- Prevention of mucositis can be helpful with use of:
    - Cryotherapy.
    - Palifermin.
    - Low level laser therapy (Photobiomodulation).

- **Oral infection**
    - Pockets of infection should be drained and eliminated.
    - Periodontitis should be aggressively addressed.
    - Caries should be aggressively managed.
    - Abscesses should be drained and treated.
    - Judicious use of antibiotics when deemed necessary.

- **Salivary gland dysfunction and xerostomia**
    - Little can be done to prevent salivary gland dysfunction with head and neck radiation.
    - Maintain good hydration.
    - Reduction of sucrose intake.
    - Oral hygiene and dental self-care.
    - Monitor for occurrence of oral candidiasis.
    - Mouth moisturizers such as Xero-Lube or Oralube can be used for rinsing.
    - Lemon-glycerin swabs are helpful.
    - Use of muscarinic agonist to stimulate saliva production:
        - Pilocarpine 5 mg three times a day.
        - Cevimeline 30 mg three times a day.

- **Infectious complications**
    - Encourage aggressive oral hygiene and provide a careful instruction of home care.
    - Judicious use of antibiotics, anti-fungal or anti-viral when indicated.

- **Oral candidiasis**
    - Nystatin suspension (400,000 to 600,000 units) four times a day; swish and swallow.
    - Use of clotrimazole troches 10 mg, up to five times a day.

- **Reactivation of herpes simplex virus**
  - Topical anti-viral when indicated:
    - Acyclovir topically every 3 hours as needed.
  - Systemic antiviral when indicated:
    - Acyclovir 200 mg five times a day for 5 days.
    - Valacyclovir 1 g twice a day for 5 days.

- **Radiation caries**
  - Encourage aggressive oral hygiene and provide a careful instruction of home care.
  - Fluoride gel applied daily, can be administered using a customized tray.
  - Fluoride rinses daily.

- **Osteoradionecrosis**
  - This complication poses problems with extractions and implants.
  - Highest risk: extractions or implants during radiation therapy should be avoided.
  - Elevated risk: 12 months or more after radiation therapy.
  - Management of osteoradionecrosis is similar to that of medication related osteonecrosis of the jaw, covered in detail in Chapter 14.

Cancer patients on head and neck radiation pose a challenge, but meticulous attention to their oral health is important for the overall health and well-being of the patient.
Attention should be paid to the oral complications associated with head and neck radiation.
Attention should also be given to patients during and after radiation therapy due to the increased risk of osteonecrosis of the jaw.

35 DENTAL EVALUATION AND MANAGEMENT OF PATIENTS ON MARROW SUPPRESSIVE CHEMOTHERAPY

INTRODUCTION

Patients on chemotherapy for a variety of cancers pose a special problem for dental professionals. There are significant oral complications that can affect dental and systemic health.

Certain chemotherapeutic regimens have impact on bone health and can cause osteonecrosis of the jaw.

The dental professional should be aware of these issues and be aggressive in management of these complications.

Patients on immunotherapy also have significant oral complications, but this was discussed in detail in Chapter 33.

1. Oral complications of chemotherapy

A number of oral complications have been causally linked with chemotherapy. Preexisting poor oral health, periodontal disease and caries considerably increase these complications.

- **Mucositis**
  - **Conventional cytotoxic chemotherapy** is typically administered in cycles.
    - Mucositis can occur within 3-5 days after chemotherapy.
    - Mucositis is generally self-limited.
    - It typically begins to improve within 3-4 days after its appearance.
    - Usually completely healed in 14 days.
  - Mucositis can also occur with **molecularly targeted chemotherapy,** but the symptoms tend to be milder.
  - Mucositis can be graded to reflect severity of involvement **(Table 35.1).**

TABLE 35.1 Grading of severity of mucositis

Grade	Description
0	No oral mucositis
1	Erythema and soreness
2	Ulcers, able to eat solid food
3	Ulcers, but requires liquid diet
4	Ulcers, unable to tolerate solid or liquid diet

- Infectious complications
  - Altered mucosal membrane due to chemotherapy can result in entry of pathogens into the bloodstream, causing systemic complications.
  - Altered immune response due to chemotherapy can increase the risk of periodontitis, caries and dental abscesses.
- Oral candidiasis
  - Candida is a common superinfection in patients with mucositis.
  - Aggressive treatment is necessary to prevent seeding of the bloodstream from this source.
- Reactivation of herpes simplex virus

  Patients with pre-existing oral herpes simplex virus are prone to reactivation during chemotherapy.
- Salivary gland dysfunction
  - Xerostomia can be a complication of chemotherapy.
  - Xerostomia can result in development of caries.
  - Xerostomia can promote oral infection.

2. Prophylactic oral care in patients on chemotherapy

If feasible, a comprehensive oral examination should be carried out before initiation of chemotherapy.

Aggressive preventive oral care has been important in preventing oral complications when chemotherapy is initiated.

Scaling and root planning, treatment of caries and endodontic therapy should be undertaken. Aggressive management of pulpal, periapical disease and periodontal disease should be done when feasible.

Unsalvageable teeth should be extracted.

It is also understood that prophylactic oral care may not be feasible because of time constraints. Nonetheless, as much preventive oral care as can be done should be undertaken.

3. Management of oral complications of chemotherapy

- **Mucositis**
  - Usually self-limited and does not require treatment.
  - Treatment, when indicated, can consist of:
    - "Miracle mouthwash": topical anesthetics (lidocaine) may be combined with an antacid suspension with or without nystatin in a cocktail.
    - Doxepin rinse.
    - Benzydamine rinse: a nonsteroidal anti-inflammatory agent given as an oral rinse.
    - Mucoadhesive hydrogel can be used as a palliative barrier over injured mucosa.
    - Palifermin may accelerate epithelial restoration.

- **Prevention of mucositis can be helpful with use of:**
  - Cryotherapy.
  - Palifermin.
  - Low level laser therapy (Photobiomodulation).

- **Oral infection**
  - Pockets of infection should be drained and eliminated.
  - Periodontitis should be aggressively addressed.
  - Caries should be aggressively managed.
  - Abscesses should be drained and treated.
  - Judicious use of antibiotics when deemed necessary.

- **Salivary gland dysfunction**
  - Maintain good hydration.
  - Oral hygiene and dental self-care.
  - Monitor for occurrence of oral candidiasis.
  - Use of muscarinic agonist:
    - Pilocarpine.
    - Cevimeline.

4. Specific chemotherapeutic agents and risk of osteonecrosis of the jaw

Some chemotherapeutic agents pose specific problems with increased risk of osteonecrosis of the jaw.

- **Anti-angiogenic agents**

  Anti-angiogenic agents are increasingly used for treatment of solid tumors (Table 35.2). Solid tumors produce a vascular endothelial growth factor (VEGF) that promotes vascular growth and blood supply to the tumor. The identification of the VEGF permits the manufacturing of VEGF inhibitors, which will hamper tumor growth by interfering with its vascular supply. Tyrosine kinase inhibitors. such as sunitinib and sorafenib, and monoclonal antibodies to VEGF (bevacizumab) are now in clinical use. Unfortunately, these agents have been associated with osteonecrosis of the jaw, likely due to their interference with the growth of new vasculature necessary for healing.

The increasing use of anti-angiogenic agents in chemotherapy is making it important not to overlook this patient population.

TABLE 35.2 Anti-angiogenic agents with risk of osteonecrosis of the jaw

VEGF inhibitors
Tyrosine kinase inhibitors
› Sunitinib (Sutent)
› Sorafenib (Nexavar)
Monoclonal antibodies to VEGF
› Bevacizumab (Avastin)

- **High dose bisphosphonates**

Bisphosphonates are important in the management of primary bone cancer, such as multiple myeloma, or metastatic bone disease (Table 35.3). They are particularly helpful in the management of bone pain in cancer patients.

In these instances, the doses prescribed are considerably higher than what would be prescribed for osteoporosis. Consequently, it is not unexpected that the incidence of osteonecrosis of the jaw is also considerably higher.

It is therefore important to identify these patients and implement aggressive preventive measures in these patients.

TABLE 35.3 High dose bisphosphonates associated with risk for osteonecrosis of the jaw

Cancer patients: **IV bisphosphonates**
Zoledronic acid (Zometa) Pamidronate (Aredia) Clodronate (Bonefos)
Significant risk Incidence 0.8-6.7%

- **High dose RANK-L inhibitors**
  RANK-L inhibitors are occasionally used for bone cancer and metastatic bone cancer. The doses are considerably higher, and they have also been associated with osteonecrosis of the jaw **(Table 35.4).**

TABLE 35.4 RANK-L inhibitor associated with risk for osteonecrosis of the jaw

Cancer patients: RANK-L inhibitor
Denosumab (Xgeva) › for reducing skeletal related events in metastatic bone disease › usually administered monthly › do not bind to bone › effect on bone remodeling diminished within 6 months of cessation of therapy **Significant risk**

Cancer patients on chemotherapy pose a challenge, but meticulous attention to their oral health is important for the overall health and well-being of the patient.
Attention should be paid to the oral complications associated with chemotherapy.
Attention should also be given to patients on chemotherapeutic agents that increase the risk of osteonecrosis of the jaw.

36 DENTAL EVALUATION AND MANAGEMENT OF THE PATIENT WITH HUMAN IMMUNODEFICIENCY VIRUS (HIV)

INTRODUCTION

Human immunodeficiency virus (HIV) is a viral infection that attacks the human immune system. It can result in acquired immunodeficiency syndrome (AIDS), where the immune system is markedly compromised with resultant infections and certain cancers. The disease is usually transmitted through sexual intercourse but can be transmitted through needles and syringes, maternal transmission or breastfeeding.

Fortunately, with aggressive antiretroviral therapy, utilizing combinations of drugs, viral replication can be suppressed, minimizing the impact on the immune system and reducing the risk of developing AIDS-related complication.

With the use of universal precautions, transmission from patient to the dental professional is unlikely. However, it is important to understand the impact of the disease on infection, including odontogenic infections. It is also important to understand the potential of drug-drug interactions from medications prescribed by the dental professional on patients on the antiretroviral therapy.

1. Dental evaluation of the patient with human immunodeficiency virus (HIV)

A detailed medical history should include information on the type of HIV the patient has, the severity of the disease, the degree of immunocompromise as indicated by the CD4 count and the stability of the disease on medication.

- **Medical history**
  - **Type of HIV:** the majority has HIV-1, but occasional patients from Africa may have HIV-2.

- **Degree of immunocompromise**
  - CD4 count on blood sample looking at CD4 T-helper cells.
  - Important measure of health of immune system.
  - Normal CD4 count is between 500 to 1,500.
  - The lower the CD4 count, the greater the degree of immunocompromise.
  - A CD4 count of less than 100 indicates that the patient is extremely susceptible to infection, including opportunistic infections and odontogenic infections.

- **Complications of HIV**
  - History of infection, including pulmonary infections, opportunistic infections and odontogenic infections.
  - History of certain types of cancer such as Kaposi sarcoma.

- **Complete list of medications the patient is on.**

2. Medications commonly used for seizures and their dental implication

Antiretroviral drugs have been developed to impair viral replications by literally attacking every phase of the viral life cycle. The patient with HIV is generally on combinations of these drugs to increase efficacy, to optimize synergy and to minimize side effects.

- **Nucleoside/nucleotide reverse transcriptase inhibitors**
  - HIV depends upon reverse transcription of its RNA in order to hijack the human cell's machinery to replicate.
  - By inhibiting the reverse transcriptase, these drugs would minimize viral replication.
  - These inhibitors are generally metabolized by CYP3A4 and would therefore be subject to potential drug-drug interactions.

- **Non-nucleoside reverse transcriptase inhibitors**
  - Also act at the reverse transcriptase site to minimize viral replication.
  - These inhibitors are generally metabolized by CYP3A4 and would therefore be subject to potential drug-drug interactions.

- **Protease inhibitors**
  - The virus would utilize the human machinery to make the proteins critical for its replication.
  - The protein is initially made as a long chain, and a viral protease is responsible for cutting this long chain into a functional protein.

- By using inhibitors specifically designed to impair the viral protease function, it would impair the production of functional viral proteins, thus limiting viral replication.
- These inhibitors are generally metabolized by CYP3A4 and would therefore be subject to potential drug-drug interactions.

- **Integrase inhibitors**
  - These inhibitors prevent the integration of the virus's genetic material into the host's DNA, thereby limiting viral replication.
  - These inhibitors are not metabolized by CYP3A4.

- **Entry inhibitors**
  - These drugs prevent the virus from entering the host cells.
  - These inhibitors are not metabolized by CYP3A4.

Since the patient with HIV is generally on combinations of these drugs, attention should be placed on drugs used in dentistry that are metabolized by CYP3A4.

3. Dental management of the patient with human immunodeficiency virus (HIV)

- **General principles**
  - All dental interventions should be avoided in patients with inadequate control of the disease.
  - All dental interventions should be avoided in patients with severe immunocompromise (a CD4 count less than 200).
  - All dental interventions should be avoided in patients in the midst of opportunistic infections.
  - Patients should be instructed to take all of their seizure medication on the morning of the appointment.

- **Oral health**
  - Aspiration pneumonia is a common complication in the patient with HIV, and optimizing oral health is important for the overall health of the patient with HIV.
  - Patients should be carefully instructed on home care.
  - Frequent recalls to optimize oral health.

- **Infection**
  - Infections, including odontogenic infections, are common in patients with HIV.
  - Aggressive treatment of odontogenic infections is important to prevent systemic sequelae.

- **Drug-drug interactions**
  - Although there are a lot of drugs that are metabolized via the CYP3A4 pathway, including statins, birth control pills and antacids, these are not drugs that are commonly prescribed by the dentist.
  - Azole antifungals, such as itraconazole and posaconazole, competitively inhibit CYP3A4 to cause significant drug-drug interactions.
  - Non-azole antifungals, such as fluconazole or voriconazole, are less potent inhibitors but can still cause modest drug-drug interactions.

4. Sedation dentistry for the patient with HIV

Patients with HIV may seek sedation dentistry. However, options would be limited because almost all of the commonly used benzodiazepines are metabolized by CYP3A4 and would be contraindicated in patients on antiretroviral medications.
Lorazepam, which is not metabolized by CYP3A4, can be used judiciously in this instance.

Dental interventions can be carried out in patients with HIV who have stable disease on medication and a reasonable CD4 count and are not in the midst of an opportunistic infection. Care should be taken to avoid drug-drug interactions for patients on antiretroviral therapy.

37 DENTAL EVALUATION AND MANAGEMENT OF THE PATIENT WITH CEREBROVASCULAR DISEASE

INTRODUCTION

Cerebrovascular disease can be the result of ischemia to the brain or hemorrhage into the brain. Patients with cerebrovascular accidents may have residual neurological damage that can complicate dental treatment planning. They are also on medications that can interfere with dental management.

1. Dental evaluation of the patient with a history of cerebrovascular disease

A detailed medical history should include the timing of the cerebrovascular event, the residual deficit the patient might have and the medications the patient is on.

Ischemic strokes

Neurological damage can be the result of cerebral ischemia from a variety of causes leading to hypoperfusion of a part of the brain.

- **Embolic stroke**
  - Embolic stroke can be the result of clots from the left atrial appendage.
  - Need to detail date of the stroke.
  - Extent of the deficits.
  - Residual deficits.
  - History of arrhythmia, particularly atrial fibrillation.
  - Medications they are on, particularly oral anticoagulants.

- **Thrombotic stroke involving large vessels**
  - Progressive obstruction of a large vessel (extracranial or intracranial) can result in thrombosis and cerebrovascular accident.
  - Need to detail date of the stroke.
  - History of surgery such as carotid endarterectomy to address the thrombosis.
  - Extent of the deficits.
  - Residual deficits.
  - Medications they are on, particularly anti-platelet therapy.

- **Lacunar stroke**
  - Luminal narrowing of small penetrating vessels progressing to occlusion.
  - Generally, the result of atherosclerotic plaques from history of hypertension.
  - Need to detail date of the stroke.
  - History of surgery such as carotid endarterectomy to address the thrombosis.
  - Extent of the deficits.
  - Residual deficits.
  - Medications they are on, particularly anti-platelet therapy.

- **Cerebral hypoperfusion**
  - Generally, an acute event with severe systemic hypotension causing generalized ischemia to the brain.
  - Most critical in the border zone area (Watershed infarction).
  - Need to detail date of the stroke.
  - Extent of the deficits.
  - Residual deficits.
  - Medications they are on, particularly anti-platelet therapy.

Cerebral hemorrhage

Cerebrovascular accidents can be the result of bleeding into the brain. This can be the result of trauma, anticoagulation therapy, bleeding diathesis or spontaneous bleeding without identifiable cause.

- **Traumatic**
  - Need to detail date and extent of traumatic brain injury.
  - History of surgery to decompress hemorrhage.
  - Residual deficits.
  - Medications they are on.

- **Spontaneous hemorrhage**
  - Long standing hypertension can lead to spontaneous hemorrhage.
  - Amyloid angiopathy can result in spontaneous hemorrhage.

- In some instances, hemorrhage may be the result of anti-coagulation or anti-platelet therapy.
- Need to detail date and extent of traumatic brain injury.
- History of surgery to decompress hemorrhage.
- Residual deficits.
- Medications they are on.

2. Medications for cerebrovascular disease

- **Embolic stroke**
  - Patients would be on anticoagulation.
  - Direct oral anticoagulants:
    - Dabigatran
    - Apixaban
    - Rivaroxaban
    - Edoxaban
    - Betrixaban
  - Coumadin

- **Thrombotic stroke involving large vessels**
  - Aggressive control of blood pressure.
  - Aggressive control of lipid profile.
  - Anti-platelet therapy.

- **Lacunar stroke**
  - Aggressive control of blood pressure.
  - Aggressive control of lipid profile.
  - Anti-platelet therapy.

- **Cerebral hypoperfusion**
  - Titrating blood pressure control.
  - Aggressive control of lipid profile.
  - Aspirin.

3. Dental management of the patient with a history of cerebrovascular disease

The dental professional should plan dental intervention with the understanding of the impact that the cerebrovascular stroke might have on dental treatment planning, the oral complications from the medications the patient is on and the potential of drug-drug interactions in medications the dentist might prescribe.

General principles

Routine dentistry including dental hygiene, simple endodontic procedures and extractions can take place 30 days after the acute event.

Elective dental surgery should be avoided within the first 6 months after an acute cerebrovascular event. This would allow the patient the optimal time to recover.

- **Embolic stroke**
  - The risk of recurrent embolization in patients with non-valvular atrial fibrillation can be estimated by evaluating all of the risk factors to arrive at a CHAD-S score (Congestive heart failure, Hypertension, Age >75, Diabetes mellitus, Stroke). The higher the CHAD-S score, the higher the risk of recurrent clots. Therefore, any thought of transient disruption of the anticoagulation must be taken in this context in consultation with the patient's physician.
  - **It is generally not necessary to interrupt anticoagulation.**
  - In instances where excessive bleeding is a concern, **minor modifications** can be done in consultation with the patient's physicians to balance the risk of embolization against the risk of excessive bleeding from the dental procedures.
  - For patients on Coumadin, it is generally not necessary to discontinue the medication. One should determine the PT/INR within 3 days of the procedure. If this PT/INR is in the high therapeutic range, it might be reasonable, in consultation with the patient's physician, to hold one dose on the night prior to the procedure to minimize excessive bleeding.
  - For patients on direct oral anticoagulants, in consultation with the patient's physician, hold the doses of medication the night before and the morning of the procedure with the intent to resume anticoagulation the night after the procedures.

- **Thrombotic stroke involving large vessels**
  - It is generally not necessary to interrupt single anti-platelet therapy.

- **Lacunar stroke**
  - It is generally not necessary to interrupt single anti-platelet therapy.

- **Cerebral hypoperfusion**
  - Titrating blood pressure control, taking care to avoid hypotension.
  - It is generally not necessary to interrupt single anti-platelet therapy.

Understanding the cause of the cerebrovascular strokes, the extent of the compromise and the medications that patient is on will allow for optimal planning of dental procedures. Modification of the medications they are on should always be made in consultation with the patient's physician.

38 DENTAL EVALUATION AND MANAGEMENT OF THE PATIENT WITH SEIZURE DISORDER

INTRODUCTION

Patients with seizure disorder pose a special challenge for the dental professionals with respect to dental treatment planning and management. The goal is to minimize situations where one might provoke a seizure and to avoid drug-drug interactions with the medications the patient may be on.

1. Dental evaluation of the patient with seizure disorder

A detailed medical history should include the type of seizure the patient has, the stability of the disease on medication and whether stress is a precipitant of the seizures. The date of onset of seizures and the medications the patient is taking are important for the optimal dental management.

The patient should be asked specifically if stress (including the stress of being in a dental chair) would precipitate a seizure.

There are different types of seizures, which are managed with different medications. The goal of the medications is to minimize the occurrence of seizures, reduce the side effects of the drugs used and optimize the patient's quality of life.

- **Focal seizures**
  - Focal area of brain as an irritable focus.
  - Seizures involving a certain body part only.
  - Patient may not have alteration of consciousness.

- **Generalized seizures**
  - Generalized tonic-clonic motion involving the entire body.
  - Patient has loss of consciousness.
  - Patient's mental status recovers slowly after the event.

- **Absence spells**
  - Transient vacant staring spells lasting 10-30 seconds.
  - Triggers may include flashing lights or hyperventilation.

- **Seizures as a result of traumatic brain injury**
  - Depending on the extent of traumatic brain injury, the seizures may be focal or generalized.

- **Seizures as a result of a brain tumor**
  - Depending upon the extent of the involvement of the tumor, the seizures may be focal or generalized.

In short, although different seizure medications may be prescribed for different clinical scenarios, certain medications are commonly used:

- Levetiracetam
- Lamotrigine
- Valproate
- Topiramate

Older medications such as phenytoin and phenobarbital are no longer used.

2. Medications commonly used for seizures and their dental implication

There are mild oral complications associated with drugs commonly used to manage seizure disorders.

The older drugs such as phenytoin and phenobarbital are seldom prescribed now; they can cause significant gingival hyperplasia.

- **Levetiracetam**
  - Mild xerostomia.
  - Rare instances of gingival hyperplasia.

- **Lamotrigine**
  - Xerostomia is a common side effect.
  - Mild gingival hyperplasia.

- **Valproate**
  - Mild xerostomia.
  - Mild gingival hyperplasia.

- **Topiramate**
  - No reports of xerostomia or gingival hyperplasia.

3. Dental management of the patient with seizure disorder

- **General principles**
  - All dental interventions should be avoided in patients with inadequate control of their seizures.
  - Patients should be instructed to take all of their seizure medication on the morning of the appointment.
  - Schedule the first morning appointment, at the time when the seizure medications should be at its maximal efficacy.

- **Gingival hyperplasia**
  - The major dental consideration for patients on seizure medications is maintenance of periodontal health. Because inflammation is likely to exacerbate gingival changes, aggressive oral hygiene and frequent professional maintenance are critical.
  - When possible, margins of fixed restorations should be placed supragingivally.
  - Patients should be carefully instructed about home care.

- **Xerostomia**
  - Maintain good hydration.
  - Reduction of sucrose intake.
  - Oral hygiene and dental self-care.
  - Monitor for occurrence of oral candidiasis.
  - Mouth moisturizers such as Xero-Lube or Oralube can be used for rinsing.
  - Lemon-glycerin swabs are helpful.
  - Use of muscarinic agonist to stimulate saliva production in severe cases:
    - ❑ Pilocarpine 5 mg three times a day.
    - ❑ Cevimeline 30 mg three times a day.

4. Sedation dentistry for the psychiatric disorder

Because stress can sometimes reduce seizure threshold, patients with seizure disorder may seek sedation dentistry.

However, patients should be clinically stable prior to consideration of sedation dentistry.

Medication regimen that can be used for sedation is discussed in Chapter 45.

39 DENTAL EVALUATION AND MANAGEMENT OF THE PATIENT WITH PSYCHIATRIC DISEASE

INTRODUCTION

Anxiety and depression are common disorders globally. Bipolar disease and psychosis are less common. A fair number of patients seeking dental care can be on medications that can affect their mental status. It is important to understand how the psychiatric disease can affect dental treatment planning. It is also important to know the dental implications of the psychoactive drugs, as they might affect planned dental interventions.

1. Dental evaluation of patients with psychiatric history

A detailed medical history should include a psychiatric history and the medications the patient is on.

- **Anxiety**
    - Degree of anxiety.
    - Duration of anxiety.
    - Medications prescribed.
    - History of panic attacks.

- **Depression**
    - Degree of depression (minor versus major).
    - Unipolar versus bipolar.
    - Duration of depression.
    - History of treatment, including medications.
    - Need for electroconvulsive therapy (ECT).

- **Bipolar disease**
  - Severity of disease.
  - Frequency of mania.
  - Medications prescribed.

- **Psychosis**
  - Severity of disease.
  - Medications prescribed.
  - History of hospitalizations.

Understanding the type of psychiatric illness the patient has and the medications they are prescribed is important for effective dental treatment planning and management.

2. Medications with psychoactive properties

A large number of medications are now used for the management of patients with psychiatric disorders. The most common ones are discussed in this section with the intention of highlighting their potential impact on dental treatment planning and management.

- **Anti-anxiety agents**
  - The major anti-anxiolytic agents prescribed belong to the benzodiazepine family.
  - It is critical to know the dose of the agents used so as to optimize dental treatment planning.
  - It is also important to know if the patient has panic attacks and the medication the patient is on for such attacks.

- **Antidepressants**
  - Selective serotonin reuptake inhibitors (SSRIs) now form the mainstay of management of depression.
  - Norepinephrine-dopamine reuptake inhibitors (NDRIs) are increasingly prescribed.
  - Serotonin modulators are sometimes prescribed.
  - Atypical antidepressants are sometimes prescribed.
  - Not infrequently, combinations of drugs may be used.
  - Older first-generation medications, such as the tricyclic antidepressants and monoamine oxidase inhibitors, are less commonly used.

- **Medications for bipolar disease**
  - First-line medications
    - Quetiapine
    - Lurasidone

- Second-line medication
  - Valproate
- Third-line medications
  - Lamotrigine
  - Olanzapine
  - Carbamazepine
  - Aripiprazole
  - Lithium: a traditional therapy, but its use is decreasing due to concerns about long-term nephrotoxicity.
- Not infrequently, combination therapy may be necessary to manage bipolar disease.

- **Antipsychotic medications**

Fortunately, psychosis and schizophrenia are uncommon psychiatric conditions. A large number of drugs are now prescribed for these conditions. Only the most common ones are listed in this section.

- First general antipsychotics: blockade of brain dopamine D2 receptors
  - Fluphenazine
  - Haloperidol
  - Chlorpromazine
  - Loxapine
  - Perphenazine
- Second generation
  - Aripiprazole
  - Clozapine
  - Olanzapine
  - Quetiapine
  - Risperidone

3. Dental management of the patient with psychiatric disorder

The dental professional should plan dental interventions with the understanding of the impact that the psychiatric condition might have on dental treatment planning, the oral complications from the medications the patient is on and the potential of drug-drug interactions with any medications the dentist might prescribe.

- **Anti-anxiety agents**
  - Mild xerostomia can be associated with benzodiazepine use.
  - Mild bruxism can be associated with benzodiazepine use.
  - Need to be judicious with use of opioids for pain management in view of increased central nervous system side effects, particularly oversedation.

- Anxious patients often seek sedation dentistry. Care should be exercised in sedating patients already on benzodiazepines.
- Benzodiazepines are the mainstay of oral conscious sedation; need to avoid oversedation.

● **Antidepressants**

- Xerostomia is common in patients on antidepressants.
- Bruxism is common in patients on antidepressants.
- Some of the SSRIs, such as sertraline and paroxetine, can cause mild gingival hyperplasia.
- SSRIs may increase the risk of osseointegrated implant failure.
- SSRIs may increase risk of halitosis.
- SSRIs can cause sore and burning tongue.
- SSRIs can cause dysgeusia.
- Need to be judicious with use of opioids for pain management in view of increased central nervous system side effects, particularly oversedation.
- Patients with depression may also seek sedation dentistry. Care should be exercised in these patients to avoid oversedation.

● **Medications for bipolar disease**

- Xerostomia is a common side effects of the major medications used in management of bipolar disease: this can lead to dental caries, gingivitis, gum recession, glossitis and stomatitis.
- Bruxism is also a common side effect of medications for treatment of bipolar disease.
- Tricyclics may accentuate the effects of vasoconstrictors; limit the use of epinephrine.
- Monoamine oxidase inhibitors can accentuate the effects of vasoconstrictors, limit the use of epinephrine.
- Need to be judicious with use of opioids for pain management in view of increased central nervous system side effects, particularly oversedation.
- Patients with bipolar disease may also seek sedation dentistry. Care should be exercised in these patients to avoid oversedation.

● **Antipsychotic medications**

- Xerostomia is a common side effects of the major medications used in management of psychosis.
- Bruxism is also a common side effect of medications for treatment of psychosis.
- Many of the antipsychotic medication can cause orthostatic hypotension. Care should be taken when getting the patient out of the dental chair.

- Need to be judicious with use of opioids for pain management in view of increased central nervous system side effects, particularly oversedation.
- Patients with psychosis may also seek sedation dentistry. Care should be exercised in these patients to avoid oversedation.

4. Sedation dentistry for the psychiatric disorder

Patients with psychiatric disorders often seek sedation dentistry. The patient needs to be cooperative and have their psychiatric condition well-controlled in order to be considered for sedation.

Sedation may take the forms of nitrous oxide, mild or moderate oral conscious sedation or advanced sedation with oral and IV techniques described in Chapter 45.

Sedation drugs should be carefully titrated down to avoid drug-drug interactions and oversedation.

The patient's physician should be consulted to optimize the use of sedation techniques.

40 DENTAL EVALUATION AND MANAGEMENT OF THE PATIENT WITH SYSTEMIC LUPUS ERYTHEMATOSUS

INTRODUCTION

Systemic lupus erythematosus (SLE) is a chronic autoimmune disease with involvement of multiple organs including skin, joints, kidneys, heart, lungs and brain.
Patients with SLE present a challenge to the dental professional who should be aware of the diverse organ systems that may be involved, the compromise immune status and the medications the patients may be on as well as their impact on dental care.

1. Dental evaluation of the patient with systemic lupus erythematosus

A detailed medical history should include the extent and severity of SLE, the organ systems involved, the medications the patient is on and the stability of the disease on medication.

- **Medical history**
  - Duration of the disease.
  - Clinical manifestation of the disease.
  - Organ systems involved, specifically inquiring about:
    - Kidney function.
    - Cardiac involvement.
    - Brain involvement.

- **Medications the patient may be taking**
  - Hydroxychloroquine: commonly prescribed to manage skin disease and joint pain.

- Non-steroidal anti-inflammatory drugs: for joint pain and inflammation.
- Corticosteroids: generally reserved for acute flares and are used for short durations.
- Immunosuppressive: generally used to spare excessive use of steroids:
    - Azathioprine
    - Mycophenolate mofetil
    - Methotrexate
    - Cyclophosphamide

2. Dental management of the patient with systemic lupus erythematosus

There are mild oral complications associated with drugs commonly used to manage patients with SLE.

- **General oral care**
    - Patient should be instructed on home care.
    - All dental interventions should be avoided in patients with inadequate control of their disease.
    - Patients should be instructed to take all of their medications on the morning of the appointment.
    - Frequent recalls.

- **Immune compromise**
    - All patients with SLE have compromised immune system.
    - This would be accentuated in patients on medications that can further compromise their immune status.
    - Patients are therefore more prone to infection and attention to their oral health is important.
    - Careful attention to caries.
    - Careful attention to periodontal disease.
    - Judicious use of antibiotics when deemed appropriate.

- **Patients with SLE and renal involvement**
    - Specifics about the extent of renal involvement is important in choice and dosing of commonly prescribed medications in dentistry.
    - In patients with known renal involvement, non-steroidal anti-inflammatory drugs are contraindicated and alternative options, such as acetaminophen, tramadol or opioids, should be considered for pain control.

- **Patients with SLE and cardiac involvement**
  - In a patient with known cardiac involvement, dental procedures should be done with ECG monitoring.
  - Use of vasoconstrictors should be limited to 2 carpules of epinephrine at 1:100,000 or levonordefrin at 1:20,000 concentrations.

Patients with SLE need careful assessment of extent and severity of their disease, attention to their medications and appropriate adjustments of dental intervention as dictated by specific organ involvement.

41 DENTAL EVALUATION AND MANAGEMENT OF THE PATIENT WITH RHEUMATOID ARTHRITIS

INTRODUCTION

Rheumatoid arthritis is a chronic autoimmune disease that primarily affects the joints. The immune system mistakenly attacks the synovium of the joint, resulting in inflammation, pain and eventually damage and deformity of the joint.
Although non-steroidal anti-inflammatory drugs and short courses of steroids can be used to treat acute joint inflammation, the goal of treatment involves prompt initiation of disease-modifying antirheumatic drugs (DMARD) in order to prevent destruction of the joints.

1. Dental evaluation of the patient with rheumatoid arthritis

A detailed medical history should include the extent and severity of rheumatoid arthritis, the medications the patient is on and the stability of the disease on medication.

- **Medical history**
  - Duration of the disease.
  - Clinical manifestation of the disease.
  - Stability of the disease.

- **Medications the patient may be taking during an acute flare**
  - Aggressive use of non-steroidal anti-inflammatory drugs.
  - Short course of corticosteroids.

  The goal of treatment is to get the patient on DMARD as soon as possible to prevent join destruction.

- **Disease-modifying antirheumatic drugs**
  - Methotrexate is the mainstay of therapy, usually in doses of 15-25 mg/week.
  - In instances where the patient is intolerant of methotrexate, other options include:
    - Leflunomide
    - Sulfasalazine
    - Hydroxychloroquine
  - In instances of refractory disease, biologics may be added to methotrexate therapy:
    - Tumor necrosis factor inhibitors:
      - Etanercept
      - Adalimumab
    - IL-6 inhibitors:
      - Tocilizumab
      - Sarilumab
    - JAK inhibitors:
      - Tofacitinib
      - Baricitinib
      - Upadacitinib
    - Rituximab

2. Dental management of the patient with rheumatoid arthritis

- **General oral care**
  - Patient should be instructed on home care.
  - All dental interventions should be avoided in patients with inadequate control of their disease.
  - Patients should be instructed to take all of their medications on the morning of the appointment.
  - Frequent recalls.

- **Immune compromise**
  - All patients with rheumatoid arthritis have compromised immune system.
  - This would be accentuated in patients on medications that can further compromise their immune status.
  - Patients are therefore more prone to infection and attention to their oral health is important.
  - Careful attention to caries.
  - Careful attention to periodontal disease.
  - Judicious use of antibiotics when deemed appropriate.

Patients with rheumatoid arthritis need careful assessment of extent and severity of their disease, attention to their medications and appropriate adjustments of dental intervention as dictated by specific organ involvement.

42 DENTAL EVALUATION AND MANAGEMENT OF THE PATIENT WITH SJÖGREN'S DISEASE

INTRODUCTION

Sjögren's disease is an autoimmune disease characterized by lymphocytic infiltration of the lacrimal and salivary glands with resultant dry eyes and dry mouth. The disease may occur in the absence of connective tissue disease (primary Sjögren's syndrome) or in association with it (secondary Sjögren's syndrome).

Secondary Sjögren's syndrome is associated with rheumatoid arthritis and systemic lupus erythematosus and, to a lesser extent, with scleroderma, polyarteritis, dermatomyositis.

The disease affects primarily females in their 40s to 50s. The distribution is 50:50 between primary and secondary Sjögren's syndrome. In secondary Sjögren's syndrome, the systemic manifestations generally precede xerostomia.

Diagnosis is generally suspected on clinical grounds and confirmed by documenting poor lacrimal and salivary gland secretions. About half of the patients with Sjögren's syndrome test positive for antinuclear antibodies (ANA) and antibodies to SSA/Ro antigens. In some cases, a biopsy of the lacrimal or salivary gland may be performed for diagnostic purposes.

Sjögren's syndrome may involve only the eyes and mouth but can also have extraglandular involvement and systemic manifestations.

Patients with Sjögren's disease have an increased risk of developing lymphoproliferative malignancies, including lymphoma, reticulum cell sarcoma and Waldenstrom's macroglobulinemia.

Although Sjögren's disease is rare, affecting less than 1% of the population, correct management of the oral manifestations is critical to optimize both oral and systemic health of the patient.

1. Dental evaluation of patients with Sjögren's disease

A detailed medical history should include a psychiatric history and the medications the patient is on.

- **Extent of involvement**
  - The disease may involve only the glandular tissues of the eyes and mouth.
  - The disease may involve skin, vagina and nose dryness.
  - The disease may have systemic manifestations, including fever and malaise.

- **Severity of disease**
  - Does the patient feel like their mouth is dry?
  - Does the patient have trouble swallowing solid food?
  - Is there oral bleeding?
  - Does the patient have salivary gland pain prior to eating?

- **Oral findings**
  - Xerostomia.
  - Bilateral parotid gland enlargement, with or without tenderness.
  - Atrophy of the filiform and fungiform lingual papillae.
  - Erythema of the lingual mucosa.

- **Salivary evaluation**
  - Both the quality and quantity of saliva can be assessed.
    - Normal salivary secretion should appear clear.
    - In Sjögren's syndrome, salivary secretion can appear thick and dark.
  - Salivary flow rate can be assessed by secretory sialography or scintigraphy.

- **Medications**
  - Medications the patient is on for salivary function should be noted.
  - Medications the patient is on that may accentuate xerostomia should be noted.

A thorough oral evaluation will help with management of dry mouth and optimize oral and systemic health.

2. Dental management of dry mouth in the patient with Sjögren's syndrome

All patients with dry mouth should be instructed on conservative management to enhance salivary flow or use a saliva substitute. In instances of severe symptoms, cholinergic medications may be used to stimulate salivary secretion.

- **Conservative management: stimulation of salivary flow**
  - Optimize hydration.
  - Use of sucrose-free lemon drugs.
  - Use of lemon-glycerin swabs.
  - Use of sugar-free drops.

- **Conservative management: use of a saliva substitute for palliation**
  - Use of artificial saliva.
  - Use of mouth moisturizer.
  - Use of lubricants to oral mucosa.

- **Medications to stimulate salivary flow**

  For patients with severe xerostomia that does not improve with conservative management, cholinergic medications may be prescribed to stimulate salivary flow:
  - Pilocarpine 5 mg, three to four times a day.
  - Cevimeline 30 mg, three times a day.

- **Oral health management**
  - Instructing patient on home self-care.
  - Addressing caries.
  - Addressing dental plaques.
  - Address ill-fitting dentures.
  - High suspicion for oral candidiasis.
  - Frequent recalls.

Although Sjögren's disease is rare, the evaluation and management issues apply to all causes of xerostomia, including xerostomia associated with a variety of commonly prescribed medications.

43 DENTAL EVALUATION AND MANAGEMENT OF THE PREGNANT PATIENT

INTRODUCTION

Pregnancy is a special time for the patient and can raise special concerns about dental management. Careful attention to certain aspects of management can benefit both maternal and fetal health.

1. General emphasis on oral health

Due to hormonal milieu changes during pregnancy, patients are more prone to gingivitis and gingival hyperplasia.

Increased in intra-abdominal pressure, decreased gastric emptying and reduced gastroesophageal junction sphincter tone can increase reflux, which can in turn affect the predisposition to gingivitis and gingival hyperplasia.

Rarely, pyogenic granuloma (pregnancy tumor), aggravated by plaques, can occur during pregnancy. Good oral hygiene can reduce the severity of these conditions.

- **Oral hygiene**
  - Maintaining oral hygiene is important for reducing the risk of gingivitis and periodontitis. Patients should be carefully instructed on the use of manual or powered toothbrushes, dental floss and other plaque-removal devices.

- **Dental cleaning**
  - There is no contraindication to dental cleaning during any phase of pregnancy, and patients should be encouraged to undergo dental cleaning as deemed appropriate.

2. Special considerations for dental interventions in the pregnant patient

Except for dental cleaning, all other elective dental interventions should be deferred until post-partum. However, if urgent dental intervention is necessary, there is no absolute contraindication to proceeding, with attention to minimizing the scope of the intervention and judicious use of local anesthetics, analgesics, narcotics and antibiotics.

- **Optimal timing of dental intervention**
  - The beginning of the second trimester (weeks 14–20 of pregnancy) is generally the best time for elective but necessary interventions.
  - Traditionally, the first trimester is to be avoided so as not to harm the fetus during organogenesis, although there is insufficient evidence to forbid interventions during this period.
  - During the third trimester, the growing fetus can cause special issues with positioning of the patient (see below).

- **Duration of dental intervention**

  In general, dental intervention should be kept as short as possible and should not exceed an hour.

- **Positioning of the patient in the dental chair**

  This is particularly a concern during the third trimester. When the patient is supine, the uterus may press on the inferior vena cava, impeding venous return to the heart and causing hypotension.

  The diaphragm is pushed upward and can impair oxygen saturation.

  Care should be taken to position the patient appropriately in the dental chair for interventions:
  - The patient's head should be higher than their feet.
  - A small pillow should be placed under the right hip to shift the uterus away from the vena cava in a supine patient.

- **Radiographs during pregnancy**

  Dental radiographs can be prescribed during pregnancy, as radiation exposure to the fetus is minimal.
  - Timing of radiographs
    - Teratogenicity is highest within the first 10 days after conception.
    - The critical period of fetal development is between 4 to 18 weeks after conception.
    - While it is prudent to avoid radiographs during the first trimester, they should not be forbidden if absolutely necessary, as the risk of radiation-induced teratogenicity is extremely low.

- Minimization of radiation exposure
  - Use a lead apron over the abdomen.
  - Use bitewings instead of panoramic radiographs.
  - Use high speed films.
  - Use rectangular collimation.

3. Use of drugs in the pregnant patient

All drugs should be used with consideration of their influence on fetal health. Drugs used in pregnancy have been classified according to their risk to the fetus **(Table 43.1)**.

TABLE 43.1 Risk categories for drugs used in pregnancy

A	No risk in animal and human studies Extensively used and/or for which there are reliable clinical data
B	Safe in animals; no human data OR Risk in animals; safe in human Data are insufficient in pregnant women to make solid estimation of human teratogenic risk
C	Risk in animals; no human data OR No animal or human data The pharmacological action of the drug may have undesirable effects on the fetus
D	Human data indicating risk
X	Teratogenic; contraindicated

It is important to know the risk categories of drugs commonly prescribed in dentistry to optimize the safety of the fetus.

4. Use of local anesthetic and vasoconstrictors in the pregnant patient

There is no evidence that judicious use of vasoconstrictors in commonly used local anesthetic preparations poses a concern. However, not all local anesthetics have the same effects on pregnant patients.

The commonly used local anesthetics and their associated risk categories are listed in Table 43.2.

TABLE 43.2 Risk categories of commonly used local anesthetics in pregnancy

Local anesthetics	
B	Lidocaine with or without 1:100,000 epinephrine
B	Prilocaine with or without 1:100,000 epinephrine
C	Mepivacaine (Carbocaine, Polocaine)
C	Bupivacaine (Marcaine)
C	Articaine (Septocaine)

Since most of dental interventions during pregnancy should be short, it is prudent to limit the use of Lidocaine or Prilocaine, with or without 1:100, 000 epinephrine, to 2 carpules per session.

5. Post-operative pain control in the pregnant patient

In general, non-steroidal anti-inflammatory drugs should be avoided during pregnancy. It is therefore possible that opioids may have to be used judiciously **(Table 43.3).**

TABLE 43.3 Risk categories of analgesics and opioids used in pregnancy

Analgesics	
B	Acetaminophen (Tylenol)
C/D*	Ibuprofen (Motrin, Advil)
C/D*	Naproxen (Anaprox, Naprosyn, Aleve)
B	Meperidine (Demerol) for short periods
C/D*	All other non-steroidal anti-inflammatory drugs (e.g., Celebrex, Ansaid, Lodine)
C	All codeine derivatives
C	All hydrocodone derivatives
C	All oxycodone derivatives
D	Aspirin

*Avoid use in the third trimester

It is clear that we have limited choices in use of analgesics and non-steroidal anti-inflammatory drugs in the pregnant patient and the use of meperidine may need to be considered carefully.

6. Use of antibiotics in the pregnant patient

Some of the antibiotics used in dentistry pose no problems, whereas others should be avoided, as listed in Table 43.4.

TABLE 43.4 Commonly prescribed antibiotics and their use during pregnancy

Antibiotics	
B	Amoxicillin
B	Azithromycin (Zithromax)
B	Clindamycin (Cleocin)
B	Cephalexin (Keflex), Cefadroxil (Duracef)
C	Clarithromycin (Biaxin)
D	All tetracyclines (Minocin, Doxycycline)

Elective dental interventions should be avoided in the pregnant patient until post-partum. However, if urgent dental intervention has to be undertaken, careful consideration must be given to the timing and duration of the procedures, the positioning of the patient and the proper use of local anesthetics, analgesics, opioids and antibiotics to optimize the safety of both the fetus and the mother.

44 DENTAL EVALUATION AND MANAGEMENT OF THE NURSING MOTHER

INTRODUCTION

Dental interventions can be safely carried out in nursing mothers, but special care should be taken to avoid inadvertent delivery of drugs to the baby via breast milk.

1. General guidelines for prescribing medications in the nursing mother

- **Minimizing potential risk to the nursing infant from maternal medications**
  - Avoid drug therapy when possible.
  - Use topical therapy when possible.
  - Medications that are safe for direct use in an infant of the nursing infant's age are generally safe for the breastfeeding mother.
  - Medications that are safe in pregnancy are not always safe in breastfeeding mothers.
  - Use reliable references for obtaining information on medications in breast milk.

- **Medication selection**
  - Choose medications with the shortest half-life and the highest protein-binding ability.
  - Choose medications that are well-studied in infants.
  - Choose medications with the poorest oral absorption.
  - Choose medications with the lowest lipid solubility.

- **Medication dosing**
  - Administer single daily-dose medications just before the longest sleep interval for the infant, usually after the bedtime feeding.
  - Breastfeed the infant immediately before administering the medication when multiple daily doses are needed.

2. Use of drugs in the nursing mother

All drugs should be used with careful consideration of their influence on the newborn's health. Not unusually, the risk categories for drugs used in pregnancy are also applied to the nursing mother (Table 44.1).

TABLE 44.1 Risk categories for drugs used in the nursing mother

A	No risk in animal and human studies Extensively used and/or for which there are reliable clinical data
B	Safe in animals; no human data OR Risk in animals; safe in human Data are insufficient in pregnant women to make solid estimation of human teratogenic risk
C	Risk in animals; no human data OR No animal or human data The pharmacological action of the drug may have undesirable effects on the fetus
D	Human data indicating risk
X	Teratogenic; contraindicated

It is important to know the risk categories of drugs commonly prescribed in dentistry to optimize the safety of the fetus.

3. Use of local anesthetic and vasoconstrictors in the nursing mother

There is no evidence that judicious use of vasoconstrictors in commonly used local anesthetic preparations poses a concern. However, not all local anesthetics have the same effect on the newborn of the nursing mother.

The commonly used local anesthetics and their associated risk categories are listed in Table 44.2.

TABLE 44.2 Risk categories of commonly used local anesthetics in the nursing mother

Local anesthetics	
B	Lidocaine with or without 1:100,000 epinephrine
B	Prilocaine with or without 1:100,000 epinephrine
C	Mepivacaine (Carbocaine, Polocaine)
C	Bupivacaine (Marcaine)
C	Articaine (Septocaine)

Most of dental interventions for the nursing mother should be short. It is prudent to limit the use of Lidocaine or Prilocaine, with or without 1:100, 000 epinephrine, to 2 carpules per session.

4. Post-operative pain control in the nursing mother

In general, non-steroidal anti-inflammatory drugs should be avoided for the nursing mother. It is therefore possible that opioids may have to be used judiciously (Table 44.3).

TABLE 44.3 Risk categories of analgesics and opioids used in the nursing mother

Analgesics	
B	Acetaminophen (Tylenol)
D	Ibuprofen (Motrin, Advil)
D	Naproxen (Anaprox, Naprosyn, Aleve)
B	Meperidine (Demerol) for short periods
D	All other non-steroidal anti-inflammatory drugs (e.g., Celebrex, Ansaid, Lodine)
D	All codeine derivatives
D	All hydrocodone derivatives
D	All oxycodone derivatives
D	Aspirin

It is clear that we have limited choices in use of analgesics and non-steroidal anti-inflammatory drugs in the pregnant patient and the use of meperidine may need to be considered carefully.

5. Use of antibiotics in the nursing mother

Some of the antibiotics used in dentistry pose no problems, whereas others should be avoided, as listed in Table 44.4.

TABLE 44.4 Commonly prescribed antibiotics and their use in nursing mothers

Antibiotics	
B	Amoxicillin
B	Azithromycin (Zithromax)
C	Clindamycin (Cleocin)
B	Cephalexin (Keflex), Cefadroxil (Duracef)
C	Clarithromycin (Biaxin)
D	All tetracyclines (Minocin, Doxycycline)

Elective dental interventions can be safely done in nursing mothers. However, special attention to prescribed medications is necessary to ensure the safety of the nursing infant.

45 DENTAL EVALUATION AND MANAGEMENT OF THE PATIENT SEEKING SEDATION DENTISTRY

INTRODUCTION

Sedation dentistry requires extensive special training and cannot be deployed without strict adherence to the legal requirements of each state.
All patients under sedation should have continuous monitoring of oxygen saturation, blood pressure and pulse. In appropriate circumstances, capnography or cardiac monitoring may also be necessary.

There are a variety of situations where the dental professional may be considering sedation dentistry for optimal patient care:

- Patients seeking dental care may have significant dental phobia and would benefit from sedation dentistry.
- Equally importantly, for patients with complicated medical conditions, it is often deemed that it would be safer to do dental procedures under sedation.
- In some instances, the complexity of the dental procedures may be such that sedation will provide for an easier operative environment and would achieve better outcomes.

1. Medical history and medication for patients seeking sedation

Sedation dentistry adds on another layer of complexity to the dental intervention. It is critical that the dentist has full access to all relevant medical information to ensure safe sedation.

- **Medical history**
    - Detailed history of medical conditions.

- Particular attention to airway issues, including:
  - History of smoking
  - History of COPD
  - History of CO_2 retention
  - Document Mallampati score

- **Prescribed medications**
  - Most of the benzodiazepines used in sedation are metabolized by the CYP3A4 system.
  - It is essential to carefully review all prescribed drugs for potential drug-drug interactions.

- **Over-the-counter medications**
  - Some over-the-counter medications, such as omeprazole, may have minor drug-drug interactions with drugs used for sedation.

- **Nutraceuticals and supplements**
  - Patients should be specifically asked about nutraceuticals since even something as innocuous as St. John's Wort may have minor drug-drug interactions with drugs used for sedation.

- **Grapefruit juice**
  - Contains furanocoumarin that can inactivate duodenal CYP3A4, resulting in increased benzodiazepine absorption.
  - Can increase peak drug levels by 55%.
  - The effect of a single dose of grapefruit juice stays in the system for 3-4 days, until new intestinal lining is re-established.

Meticulous attention to all of these issues is essential for safe and effective sedation dentistry.

2. Assessment of level of sedation desired

The dental professional should take into account the patient's level of anxiety, the complexity and duration of the dental intervention, and the patient's medical condition in order to gauge the appropriate level of sedation.

- **Anxiolysis**
  - The mildest level of sedation.
  - Drugs used for anxiolysis tend to be short acting and less potent.
  - However, oversedation can occur if excessive amount of sedation drug is used.

- **Minimal sedation**
  - Under minimal sedation, the patient can independently and continuously maintain their airway.
  - The patient responds normally to tactile stimulation and verbal commands.
  - Mild cognitive impairment.
  - Normal respiratory and cardiovascular function.

- **Moderate sedation**
  - The patient can maintain their airway independently.
  - The patient can respond to loud commands.
  - Normal respiratory and cardiovascular function.

- **Deep sedation**
  - **Should only be employed by professionals with significant training in IV sedation.**

3. Dental management of the patient seeking sedation

All patients under sedation should undergo continuous monitoring of oxygen saturation, blood pressure and pulse. In appropriate circumstances, capnography or cardiac monitoring may also be necessary.

- **Anxiolysis**
  - Nitrous oxide is commonly used for anxiolysis, often during the administration of local anesthetics.
  - Nitrous oxide may be used to assist during very short extension of an appointment running longer than planned.
  - Alternatively, a short-acting benzodiazepine **(Table 45.1)** may be prescribed.
    - Triazolam or Zaleplon.
    - A single dose given 30 minutes prior to the procedure.
    - No redosing.

- **Minimal sedation**
  - Proper training is important.
  - Diazepam is often given the night before the procedure.
  - A short-acting benzodiazepine is often given 30 minutes before the procedure.
    - Triazolam or zaleplon, with or without hydroxyzine may be prescribed.
  - Repeat dosing according to protocol as defined by the state's guidelines.
  - Lorazepam may be used, particularly if there is concern over CYP3A4 drug-drug interaction with the medications.

- **Moderate sedation**
  - Proper training is important.
  - Diazepam is often given the night before the procedure.
  - A short-acting benzodiazepine is often given 30 minutes before the procedure.
    - Triazolam or zaleplon with or without hydroxyzine may be prescribed.
  - Repeat dosing to titrate to level of sedation desired, according to protocol.
  - Lorazepam may be used, particularly if there is concern over CYP3A4 drug-drug interaction with the medications.

- **Deep sedation**
  - **Should only be employed by professionals with full training and certification in IV sedation.**

TABLE 45.1 Oral sedation medications

	Generic	Trade name
Short acting	Triazolam	Halcion
	Zaleplon	Sonata
Intermediate acting	Hydroxyzine	Atarax or Vistaril
	Lorazepam	Ativan
Long acting	Diazepam	Valium

4. Reversal agent for sedation dentistry

Flumazenil should be immediately available in the operatory in all patients undergoing sedation dentistry. Since the half-life of flumazenil is relatively short, one should be prepared to repeat the reversal agent 15 minutes after the first dose if the patient remains lethargic.

AUTHORS

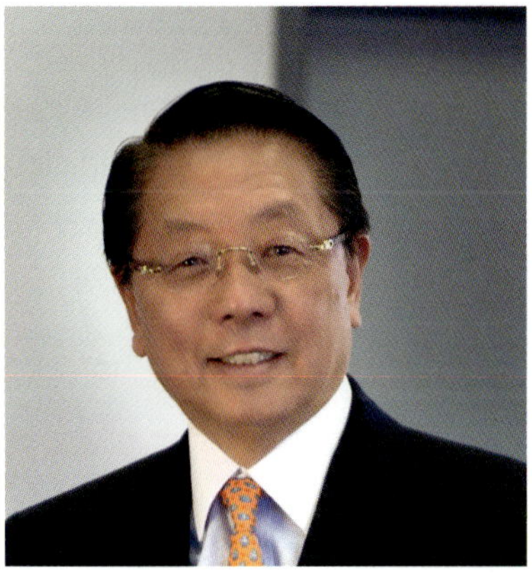

LESLIE S.T. FANG, MD, PhD

In medicine

Leslie S.T. Fang received his PhD degree in Physiology and Biophysics from the University of Illinois, Champaign-Urbana. He did his medical training at Harvard Medical School and was elected to Alpha Omega Alpha as a junior. He did his residency training at the Massachusetts General Hospital where he served as Chief Medical Resident.

He did his fellowship training in Nephrology at the Massachusetts General Hospital and is board certified in Internal Medicine and Nephrology. He has been on the staff of Massachusetts General Hospital and on the faculty of Harvard Medical School. A clinician and a teacher, he maintains an active international practice in Internal Medicine and Nephrology and is a leading teacher at Harvard Medical School. At the Massachusetts General Hospital, he served as Chief of the Walter Bauer Firm and as the Clinical Director of the Governing Board of the Medical Services Associates. He has received numerous awards for excellence in teaching from Harvard Medical School and has served and chaired the Medical Internship Selection Committee at the Massachusetts General Hospital for two decades. He has been repeatedly honored among the Best Doctors of America and Best Doctors of Boston.

He is the John R. Gallagher III and Katherine A. Gallagher Endowed Chair in Clinical Excellence at the Massachusetts General Hospital. He is the Chairman of the Leslie S.T. Fang Foundation and the GoFAR Foundation.

In dentistry

With Dr. Robert Fazio and Dr. Stephen Sonis, he is the co-author of the major textbook Principle and Practice of Oral Medicine and the Oral Medicine Secrets and has been heavily involved in the clinical teaching of Oral Medicine. With Dr. Fazio, he is the co-author of an interactive DVD on Antibiotics in Dentistry in the EndoMagic Interactive Teaching Series, which was ranked by CRA among the best product for 2003. The Ultimate Cheat Sheets was voted the Best Product of 2008-2015 by Clinician Report and is now designated a Classic in Educational Product.

He has been the featured speaker at many of the major dental meetings. He has been integrally involved in the EndoMagic course and courses at the Las Vegas Institute of Advanced Dentistry. He is involved with courses in Oral Conscious Sedation, IV Sedation, Pediatric and Teem Sedation, Sedation Solutions and Master Series with DOCS. He was voted as one of the top clinicians in Continuing Education in Dentistry by Dentistry Today.

In education

He is active in national and international medical and dental education. He teaches interactively using a case-based method and actively involves his audience in the lecture. He was in charge of the third- and fourth-year clerkship in Medicine at the Massachusetts General Hospital for over two decades. He was integrally involved in the medicine and nephrology training program and has been voted best clinical teacher in the Harvard system on seven separate occasions. He gives over 100 lectures annually on a large variety of clinical topics and has a strong following internationally.

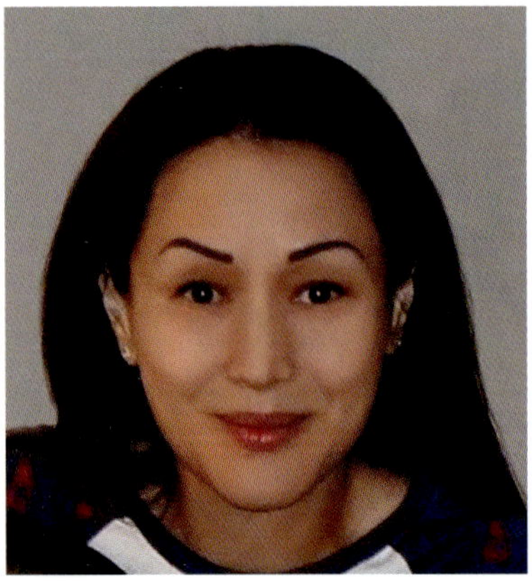

TRACEY WONG MENHALL, MSc

Tracey Menhall is a 1989 graduate from Harvard University with a degree in Economics. She received her MS degree in Asset Allocation and Portfolio Management from Massachusetts Institute of Technology. She is also a certified CPA.

She was in mutual fund consulting at Price Waterhouse and in fixed income portfolio management at Fidelity. She then worked for Medical Science Partners, the venture capital fund affiliated with Harvard Medical School.

For the past 16 years, she has been instrumental in case-based interactive learning forums and is responsible for the research and design of most of the educational material used by Leslie Fang, MD, PhD.

She is responsible for content development and production of every edition of The Ultimate Cheat Sheets. She is also the Chief Operations Officer and a Trustee for both the Leslie S.T. Fang Foundation and the GoFAR Foundation.